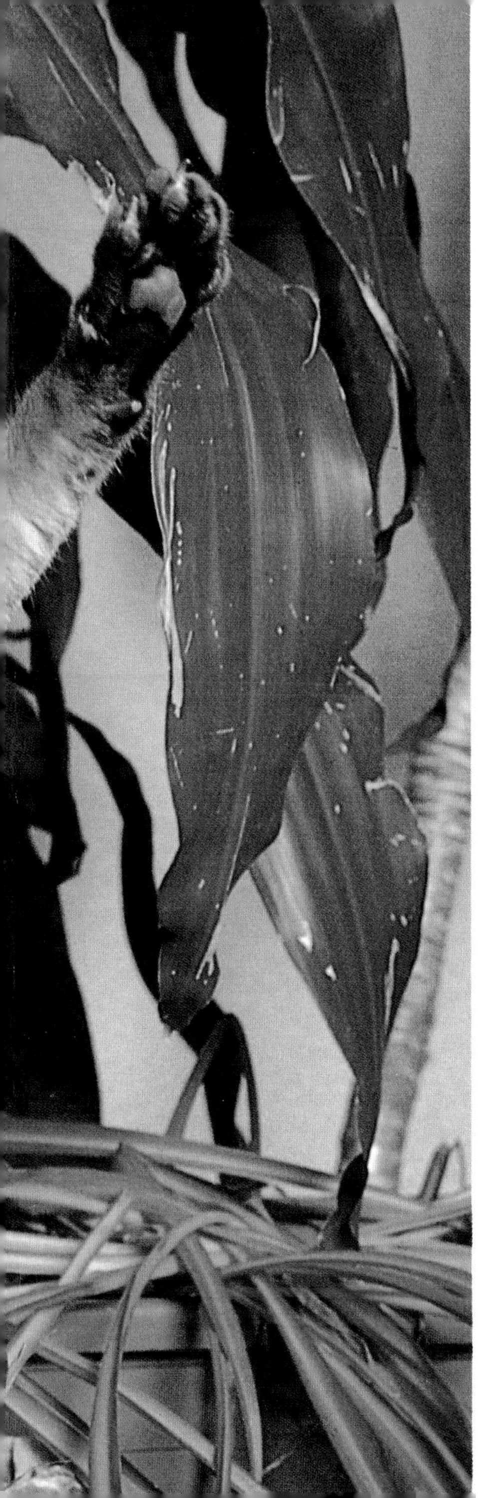

Ulrike and H. Alfred Muller

Healthy Cat, Happy Cat

A Complete Guide to Cat Diseases and Their Treatment

Contributing author:
Heidrun Gratz

Drawings by Renate Holzner and color photos by Christine Steimer and other renowned animal photographers

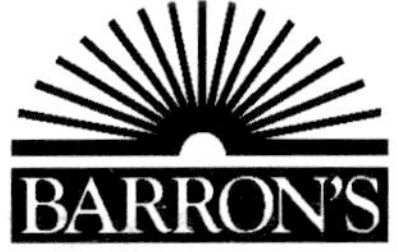
BARRON'S

Contents

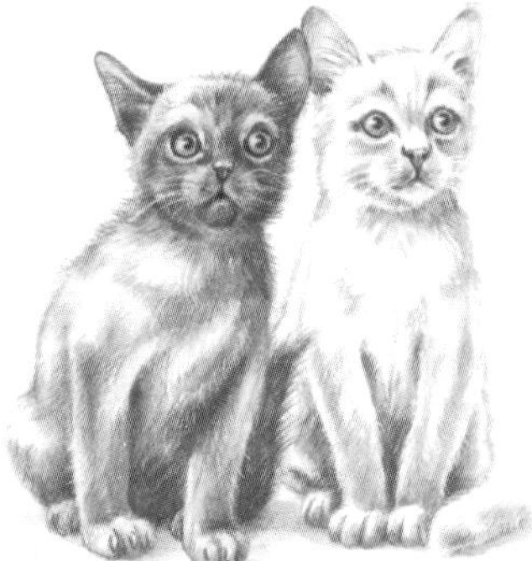

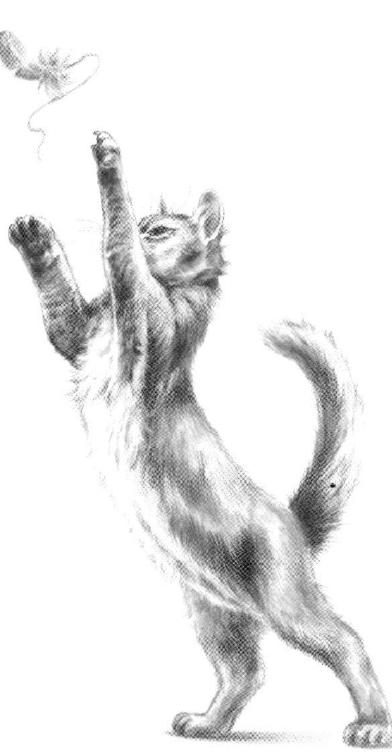

Preface

Has there been a change in your cat's behavior? Is your pet apathetic, or has it lost its appetite? These and other signs are indications of illness. This new Barron's pet owner's manual tells you what needs to be done. The Table of Symptoms will give you some clues to your cat's disease. In the disease section the most important diseases of cats are described, along with the treatments. The authors explain in precise, easy-to-understand language how you can help your sick pet yourself or how a veterinarian can help. Tips on treatment with homeopathic remedies that seem promising are also listed. Common technical terms are explained.

The basic requirements for keeping your pet healthy are the best possible living conditions and preventive care, including vaccinations. The chapter "Keeping Cats Healthy" contains all the information you need.

The how-to pages provide tips on grooming and feeding, as well as instructions for giving first aid. Photos and drawings will help you put the suggestions into action. The authors and pet editors of Barron's books wish your cat a speedy recovery.

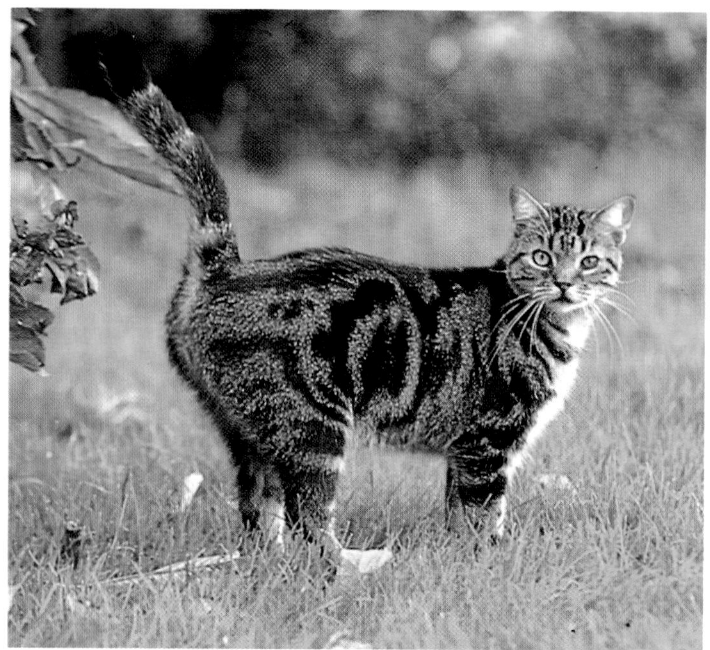

Sexually mature male cats mark their territory with their urine.

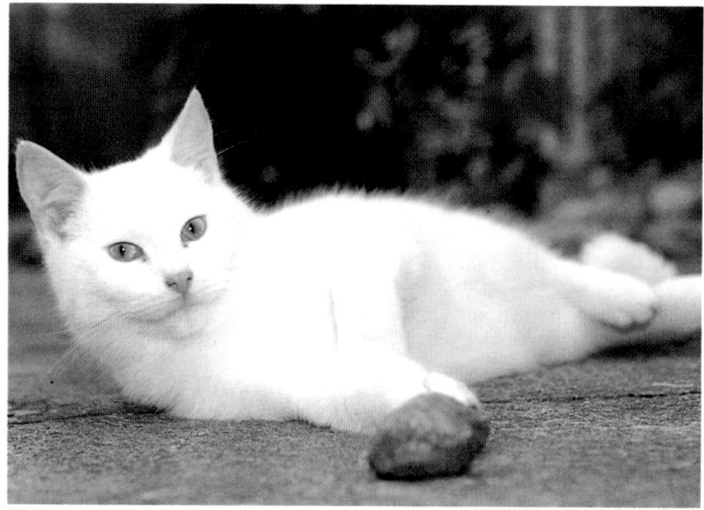

This cat watches its surroundings attentively.

Table of Symptoms

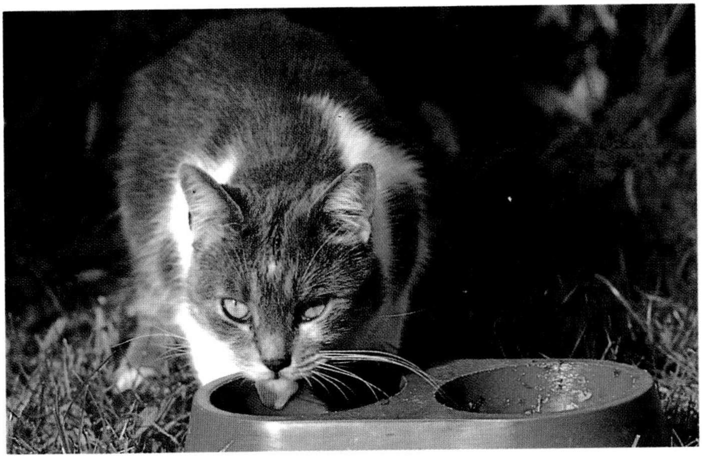

A Table of Symptoms is presented on pages 6–9. This table is intended to help you quickly track down your cat's illness. Of course, the table out of necessity is very simple and therefore cannot provide exhaustive information. Often, too, a serious disease is concealed behind an apparently innocuous health disturbance. It is always best to take your pet to a veterinarian as soon as you notice any change in its behavior or any symptoms of disease.

Cat owners usually can tell very quickly if their pets are ill, especially if pet and owner live in close contact. Knowing something about the cat's natural modes of behavior is extremely helpful. For this reason, the chapter entitled "Typical Patterns of Behavior" (see page 28) presents a profile of the average cat.

The most common symptoms of disease are apathetic behavior, neglect of grooming, dull coat, severe itching, and sudden failure to use the litter box. These symptoms, and others, are presented in the following table as well as discussed more fully in the disease section of this book (see pages 64–111).

The correct drink for cats is fresh water.

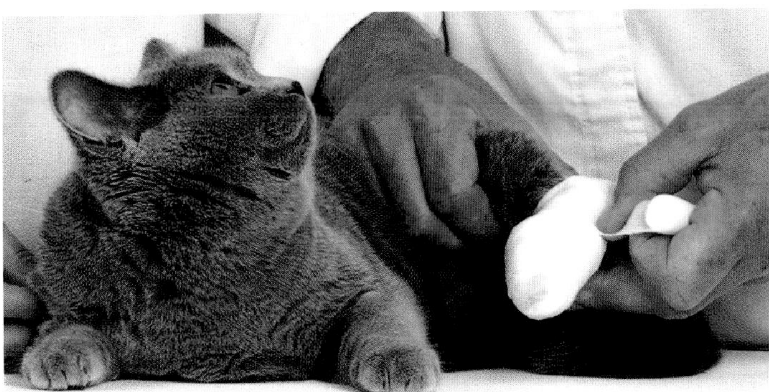

This cat patiently allows its injured paw to be bandaged.

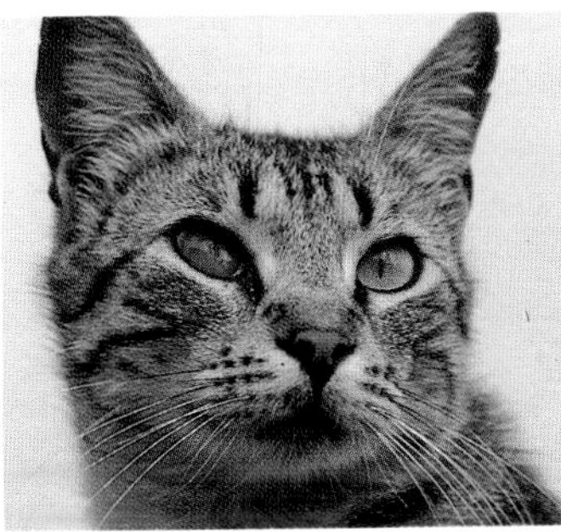

Cat with eye disease.

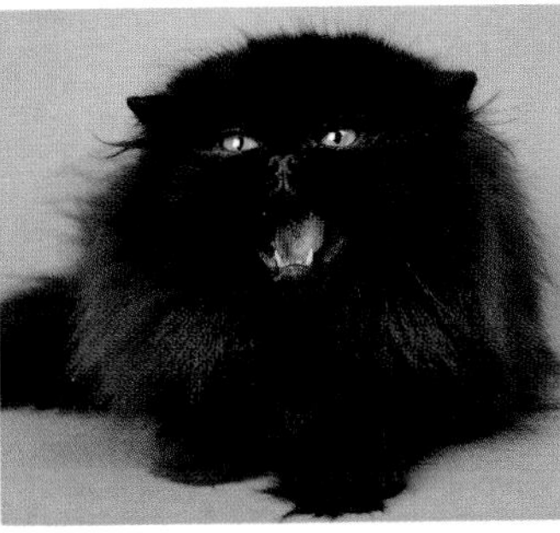

A fascinating feline face.

Quick Recognition of Diseases

Symptom	Possible Causes That You Can Correct Yourself	Cause for Alarm If These Symptoms Also Are Present
Lack of appetite	Cat is full, self-supplier catches mice or is fed by neighbors, finicky eater, unaccustomed food, heat in female cats	Behavioral abnormalities, apathy, weight loss, fever, subnormal temperature, vomiting, diarrhea or absence of stool, drooling, gagging
Large appetite	Long period without food, special stress such as pregnancy, cold weather, behavioral changes	Weight loss, obesity, drinks a great deal of water
Won't drink	High water content of food, has other sources of drinking water	Apathetic behavior, drooling
Drinks a great deal	Dry food, very dry air indoors, hot weather	Vomiting, subnormal temperature, weight loss, apathetic behavior, lack of appetite, weakness
Diarrhea	Change in diet, great excitement, stress, has drunk milk	Apathetic behavior, dehydration, weight loss, vomiting
Vomiting	Eats large amounts of food too fast, indigestible food, has eaten plant parts or hair	Repeated vomiting, apathy, fever, diarrhea, absence of stool
Bad breath	Comes from food such as fish	Drooling, pain when eating, vomiting, drinks a great deal, breath smells of urine
Straining, without passage of stool or urine	Constipation due to lack of exercise, obesity, labor in females	Prolonged straining without success, bloody stool, vomiting, some blood in urine, expression of pain, licking the tip of the penis

Possible Diagnosis	Description of Disease
Systemic infection, organic disease	Pages 80, 104
Tumors	Pages 44, 75
Infection, foreign body in digestive tract	Pages 84, 104
Rabies	Page 108
Constipation	Page 86
Diseases of oral cavity/teeth, infection	Page 68
Parasite infestation	Page 96
Hormonal disturbance	Page 77
Behavioral abnormality	Page 31
Serious infections	Page 104
Rabies	Page 108
Disease of oral cavity, foreign body swallowed or in mouth	Pages 68, 84
Kidney damage	Page 80
Diabetes, inflammation of pancreas	Pages 79, 89
Uterine infection	Page 82
Parasite infestation	Page 96
Infection, poisoning	Pages 54, 104
Disease of liver, pancreas	Page 88
Infectious diseases (such as FPL)	Page 104
Organic diseases, kidney damage	Page 80
Gastritis, poisoning	Pages 54, 86
Constipation, paralysis of the bowels	Pages 86, 87
Intestinal obstruction	Page 87
Gingivitis	Page 69
Abscess, tooth disease	Pages 68, 74
Gastritis	Page 86
Kidney damage	Page 80
Severe constipation, sluggish bowels	Page 86
Tumors	Pages 44, 75
Urinary tract infection	Page 80
Gravel, urinary calculus, or Feline Urological Syndrome (FUS)	Page 81

Symptom	Possible Causes That You Can Correct Yourself	Cause for Alarm If These Symptoms Also Are Present
Excessive or frequent urination	Has drunk a great deal, marking behavior	Cat repeatedly releases small amounts of urine, bloody urine, large amount of urine
Sneezing, coughing	Irritants in the air	Apathetic behavior, eye inflammation, nasal discharge, heavy breathing, fever, drooling, difficulty breathing, weakness
Rapid, labored breathing	Increased need for oxygen after exertion, excitement, cooling down in very hot weather	Apathy, fever, coughing, sneezing, fast heart beat, pale or blue mucous membranes, abdominal breathing
Changes in skin, hair loss, itching	Dirt, natural or delayed shedding, matted hair	Incessant scratching of head, scratching of body, localized hair loss, purulent or scaly areas, severe general disturbance
Lameness	Minor bruise or strain after accident, superficial footpad injury	Extreme, varying, or prolonged lameness, apathetic behavior
General increase in girth, localized swelling	Obesity, pregnancy	Apathetic behavior, fever, weight loss while abdomen remains large
Failure to use litter box	Marking behavior of intact animals, disturbing environmental conditions	Diarrhea, frequent straining, lameness

Possible Diagnosis	Description of Disease
Urinary tract infection, gravel, FUS	Page 81
Kidney or liver damage, diabetes	Pages 79, 80, 88
Uterine inflammation	Page 82
Feline respiratory disease complex	Page 107
Inflammation or foreign body in nose or larynx	Page 84
Respiratory disorders	Page 90
Lung congestion, heart trouble	Page 94
Respiratory tract infection	Page 91
Blood loss, anemia, shock, heart trouble	Page 95
Damage to chest cavity because of accidents	Page 93
Ruptured diaphragm	Page 93
Ear inflammation, mange, mites	Pages 68, 96, 97
Fleas, lice, mange, allergy	Pages 96, 97
Hormonal disorder, malnutrition	Pages 21, 77
Fungal infection	Page 111
Aujeszky's disease	Page 105
Injuries to locomotor apparatus	Page 70
Infections, errors in feeding	Pages 21, 104
Metabolic disorder, joint inflammation	Pages 72, 77
Injured paw	Page 71
FIP, tumors	Pages 44, 75, 104
Intestinal parasites, FIP	Pages 100, 104
Hematomas, abscesses, inflammations	Pages 67, 74, 86
Uterine infection	Page 82
Intestinal infection, urinary tract infection	Pages 81, 87
Kidney damage caused by injury or infections	Page 80

Keeping Cats Healthy

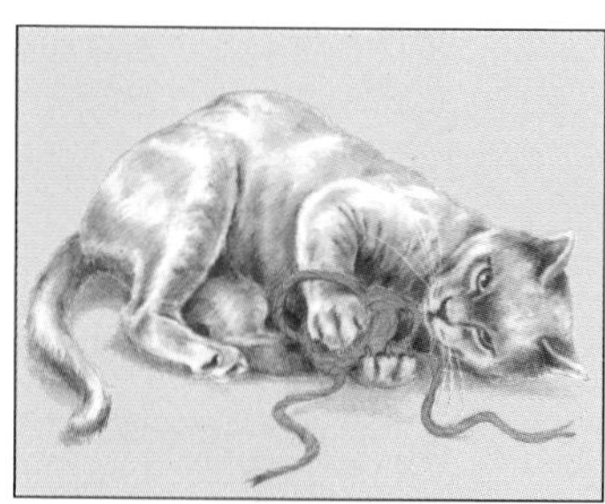

An indoor cat can have a life span as long as 20 years. For a cat to reach advanced age in good health, it needs, above all, loving care, a balanced diet, and proper grooming. The daily hour or so of cuddling and the opportunity to play with its human also contribute to a cat's well-being. By taking appropriate preventive measures, pet owners may be able to keep their cats from developing diseases.

Prevention Is Basic

A thick, glossy coat that is scrupulously licked clean several times a day, bright eyes, a good appetite, and a lively interest in everything going on around it: these are the hallmarks of a healthy cat. Cat owners can contribute a great deal to the health of their pets. Loving devotion is of prime importance, but appropriate care, a balanced diet, regular grooming, and preventive measures like vaccination and deworming are also fundamental to keeping your cat well (see "Precautionary Measures," page 23).

Indoor Cats

Cats are well suited for a life spent exclusively indoors. If a cat has not had the experience of being allowed outdoors while it was a kitten, it will certainly never miss that experience in later life. Longhaired cats such as Persians because of the nature of their coats are completely unsuited for a life that includes time outdoors.

Indoors there is substantially less risk of infection and injury. Limited activity and the decreased availability of environmental stimuli are compensated for by a safe, protected life, which cats greatly relish. The larger the house or apartment, the more varied its furnishings, and the more personal attention a cat receives from its owner, the happier the animal will feel.

A cat-correct home needs to have suitable places for a cat to rest (cabinets, upholstered furniture, special cavelike beds). Also make sure that there are no potential hazards for your pet, such as exposed electric cables, hot burners, and indigestible objects like Christmas tree icicles, plastic toys for children, or sewing needles. Don't grow poisonous plants indoors or on your balcony (hyacinth, lily of the valley, narcissus, poinsettia, primrose), and dispense with any plants on which the cat might hurt itself, such as cactuses. Do not leave detergents, household cleansers, or chemicals out in your home. A cat could be poisoned or burned if it licked these agents.

Scratching devices should be placed, if at all possible, near the cat's favorite resting places. Cats do not sharpen claws on scratching posts; when cats scratch, they are removing dead husks of claws. Appropriate types of products are scratching mats made of carpeting, corrugated cardboard wedges, scratching posts, scratching trees, or—ideal for indoor cats—scratching tree houses (available in pet stores or from mail order suppliers). It is important that scratching posts be stable and not tip

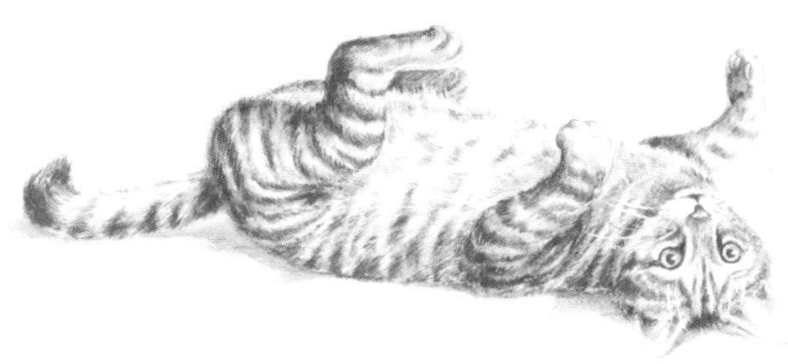

This posture is the cat's way of saying "Play with me."

over the first time the cat jumps up on them. A cat that has had such an experience will never use the scratching post again.

A place to eat, where drinking water is always available and food is put out at fixed times, is essential. It is best to serve drinking water and dry cat food in heavy, glazed, lead-free ceramic bowls that your pet cannot push around or turn over. Moist food (meat, canned cat food, mushy food) can be served in small stainless steel bowls, which are heatproof and easy to clean (see "Proper Nutrition," page 16).

The cat's litter box should be put in a place easily accessible at all times. Put it in a place where the cat will be undisturbed, not too close to its food and water bowls. Put a layer of cat litter about 2 inches (5 cm) deep in the litter box. There is no need to empty the box completely every day. With a small scoop remove only the feces and the damp spots, then add fresh litter. Once a week clean the cat box with hot water. Don't use a disinfectant: Cats dislike the odor and might find another place in your home to do their business.

Toys, including crocheted wool mice suspended from ribbons, empty cardboard boxes, tennis balls, and the cat toys

Health Check

Coat:	Thick, glossy
Skin:	Elastic, soft, and smooth
Ear canals:	Clean
Anal opening and surrounding area:	Clean
Mucous membranes:	Pink
Nostrils, eyes:	Free from accumulated secretions
Appearance of urine:	Clear, yellow
Appearance of stool:	Cylindrical in form; moist, soft consistency; dark gray to brown color
Body temperature:	100–103°F (37.8–39.2°C)
Body weight:	5–12 pounds (2.5–5.5 kg)
Pulse beats per minute:	130–140 (kittens) 110–130 (young cats) 100–120 (old cats)
Breaths per minute:	40 (kittens) 30 (young cats) 20 (old cats)

available in pet stores, provide entertainment and may keep the cat from choosing curtains or upholstered furniture to use as playthings.

A cat carrier made of plastic and equipped with a latch is a useful acquisition (see photo, page 48). A carrier is indispensable if you take the cat along on trips or have to transport your pet to the veterinarian.

Letting Your Cat Go Out

A cat that lives predominantly indoors can also be accustomed to roaming freely outdoors or going out in a fenced, escape-proof part of your yard. The cat will use its time outside to defecate and urinate, scratch trees, and—insofar as possible—engage in playing and hunting.

In addition, outdoor exercise provides the cat with interesting stimuli from the environment and toughens the cat through exposure to weather factors. You will, however, have to accept that your pet runs a greater risk of harm through infections and accidents.

If an apartment is too cramped, if a cat owner has too little time for his or her pet, or if the cat is not housebroken, outdoor exercise also can be helpful. Responsible cat owners, however, should see to it that their pets are neutered if they are going to spend time outdoors, in order to prevent unplanned offspring (see "Altering or Sterilization," page 24).

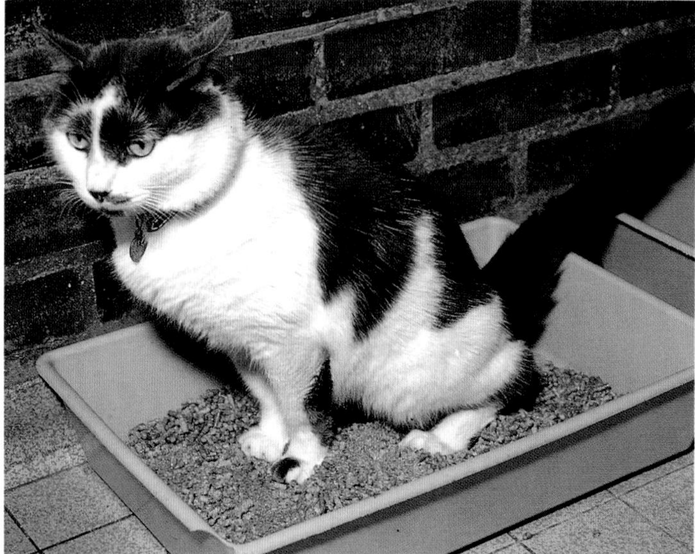

Sometime between the third and fifth weeks of life, cats begin to use a litter box.

Regular health check-ups and vaccinations, along with a balanced food supply and potential hiding places, should be provided as a matter of course.

Feral Cats

Many cats spend their entire lives outdoors. Cats' typical hunting behavior is especially prized on farms where animals are kept and where large amounts of grain and other feeds are stored. In previous times neither secure silos nor chemical agents for rodent control were available. The spread of the noxious mouse and rat populations often could be prevented only by yard cats.

On a farm feral cats' dealings with humans generally are limited to receiving some fresh milk in the cow stable. At first glance such cats appear to have a lovely life, assuming there are enough mice in the surrounding countryside and not too many cats living in the area.

Unfortunately, the real situation of feral cats often looks quite different. Many cats die of infectious diseases, become infested with parasites, are poisoned by insecticides or other substances, or are run over by cars. Moreover, cats often meet an early death, killed by a hunter's rifle bullet or by the bites of a dog. Injuries incurred during fights between tom cats are most common among feral cats, as are battles over living and hunting territories.

Feral cats are largely independent of, though not always

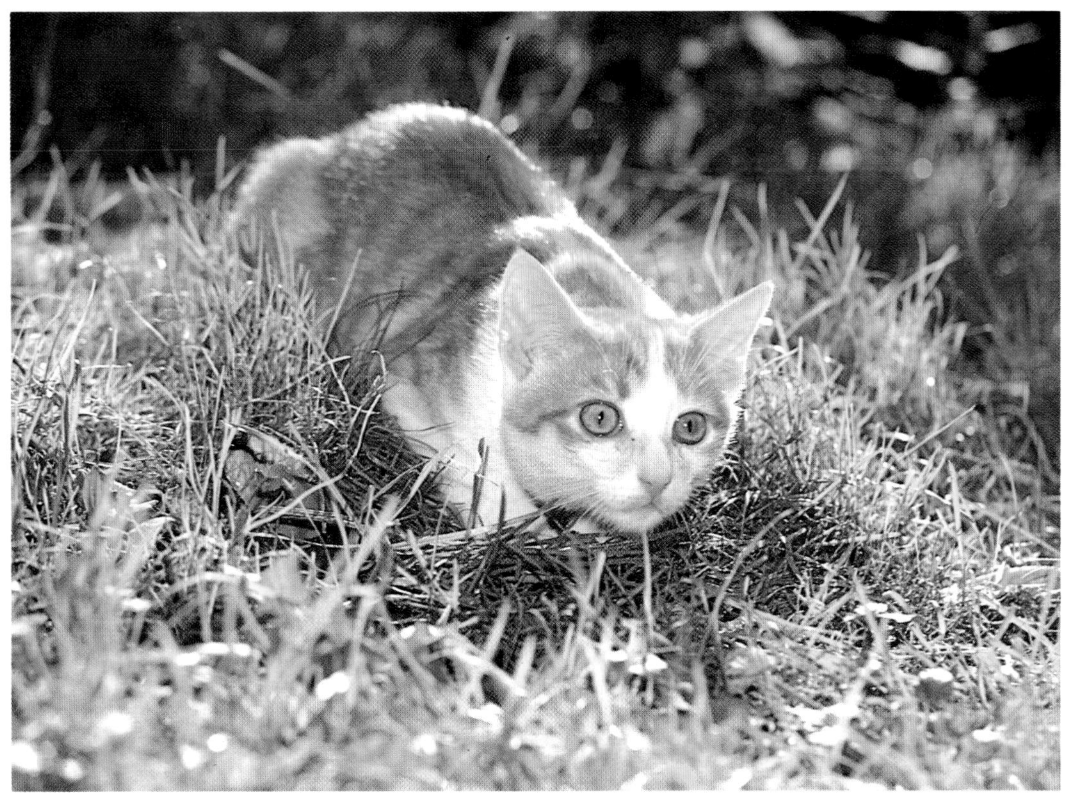

This cat is silently creeping up on a mouse. Free-roaming cats are exposed to a great many dangers, including fatal infectious diseases and injury or death from being struck by a car.

unaffected by, human conduct. They usually will accept food from people, yet they may not accept a person's presence while they eat. Feral cats are sometimes called wild cats, but they are often more wily than wild, and the more genial among them are not wild at all.

Nobody knows how many feral cats there are in this country. In 1993 a research firm in New York City conducted a survey of cat and dog owners for the Humane Society of the United States. Nearly one out of four persons surveyed (24 percent) reported that he or she fed stray cats. Some people fed one cat, some two, others three, still others more. Judging by the number of cat and dog owners in this country, that 24 percent equals 15.3 million well-intentioned people feeding 36 million feral cats.

Feeding feral cats is not as kind as it may seem. The person who feeds a feral cat is helping it to stay healthy enough to produce more feral kittens. Instead of simply putting out food for a cat, a person also should befriend that cat (or trap it in a humane trap), take the cat to the Humane Society, have it altered, and return it to its territory. Many animal shelters will lend out the traps necessary for trapping a cat that cannot be handled.

HOW-TO: Preventive Care

Comb and Brush for Coat Grooming

Shorthaired cats, as a rule, need to be brushed thoroughly at least once a week to keep them from swallowing too many dead hairs when they clean themselves (see "Constipation," page 86). The coats of longhaired cats, however, have to be groomed more frequently; otherwise, their hair easily becomes matted.

The following tools are needed for coat care:

• For short- and long-haired cats, a semiround brush with firm natural bristles or a rubber brush with nubs.

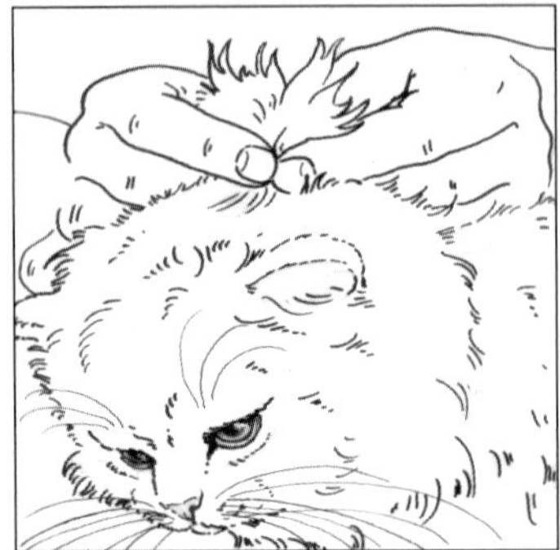

1) With your fingers carefully loosen the matted knots.

• In addition, for longhaired cats, two metal combs, one coarse-toothed and the other fine-toothed, and a dematting tool for removing knots in the coat hair.

Combing should start with the coarse-toothed metal comb. Don't forget to give the undercoat on the cat's belly and the area between its legs a thorough combing to prevent matting. Finally, use the fine-toothed comb to go over the entire coat one more time, working from head to tail. Keep an eye out for fleas (see "Cat Fleas," page 98).

Brushing ensures a glossy coat. Always brush with the lay of the coat. Most cats show their enjoyment at being brushed by purring loudly.

Bathing, in general, should only be done if your cat is extremely dirty or if bathing is part of the therapy required for treatment of a disease. Suitable moisturizing shampoos are available from your veterinarian or in pet stores.

In a room kept at a moderate temperature, carefully place the cat in a tub of warm water (86–95°F [30–35°C]). Hold the cat's front paws with one hand while washing the cat with the other hand. The head needs to stay dry. Rinse thoroughly to remove all traces of shampoo. Rub the coat thoroughly dry with a heated towel, then let the cat finish drying in a warm room.

Removing Knots of Hair

First, use your fingers to separate the knots into several small sections, then try to untangle them with a comb that has a handle. If that fails, cut through the knots with a dematting tool (available in pet stores). Guide the tip of the dematter with your finger to keep from injuring the cat's skin.

Hint: If Persian cats are not combed daily, large numbers of knots can form. Then the animals have to be clipped under general anesthesia at a veterinarian's office.

Proper Ear Care

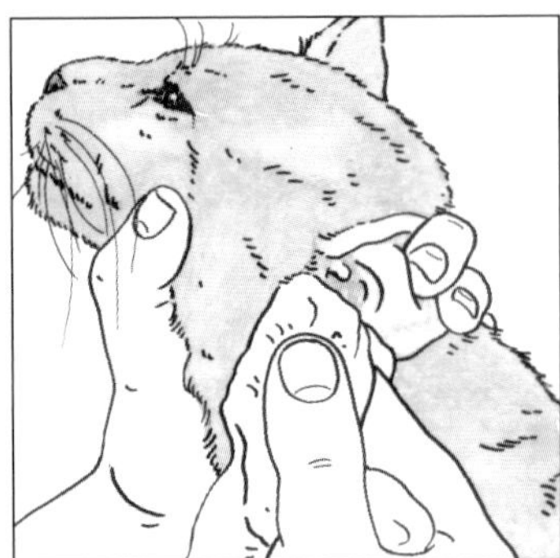

2) Clean the external ear with a tissue.

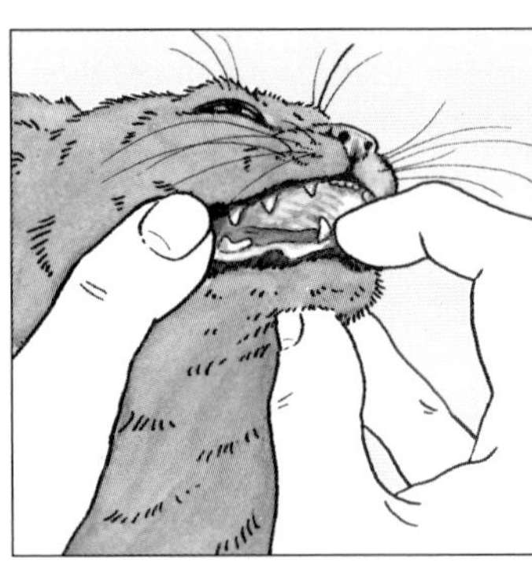

3) Check the teeth regularly for tartar build-up.

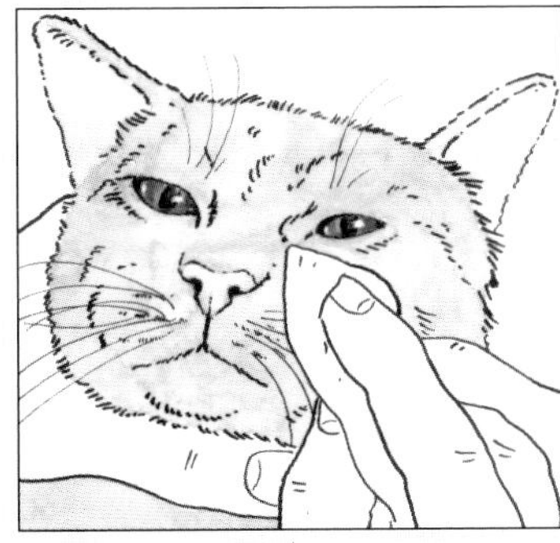

4) Remove eye secretions with a tissue.

The cat's ears have to be checked regularly. If the external ears are dirty, clean them carefully with a damp paper tissue or cotton ball. If small, dark clumps are visible and the cat shakes its head repeatedly and scratches itself frequently, you need to consult a veterinarian. Your pet could have ear mites (see page 96).

Teeth and Mouth Care

Both common domestic and purebred cats have a tendency to tartar formation and gingivitis (inflammation of the gums). For that reason it is necessary to inspect their teeth on a regular basis.

Tartar formation is promoted by overly soft food. Dry cat food and other hard components in a cat's diet offset the process somewhat. If tartar forms nonetheless, it has to be removed by a veterinarian (see page 68).

Gingivitis can develop as a result of tartar or can be caused by infections in the mouth and throat. A red border at the edge of the gums is a telltale sign. The cat also will have very bad breath (see page 69).

Eye Care

Even the eyes of healthy cats tear at times. With a soft, dampened paper tissue you can remove slight encrustations in the corners of your pet's eyes, always making sure to wipe from the eye toward the nose.

A sudden, copious flow of tears from one eye may indicate that a foreign body is present (see page 65). Only a veterinarian can remove the foreign body. Reddened eyes with a sticky yellow discharge are signs of conjunctivitis (see page 64).

Persian cats often have a constriction or obstruction of the tear ducts, resulting in watering eyes and yellow stains on the fur. Once a day, or more often if necessary, dry the tears with a clean, soft paper tissue. The veterinarian can also prescribe eye drops.

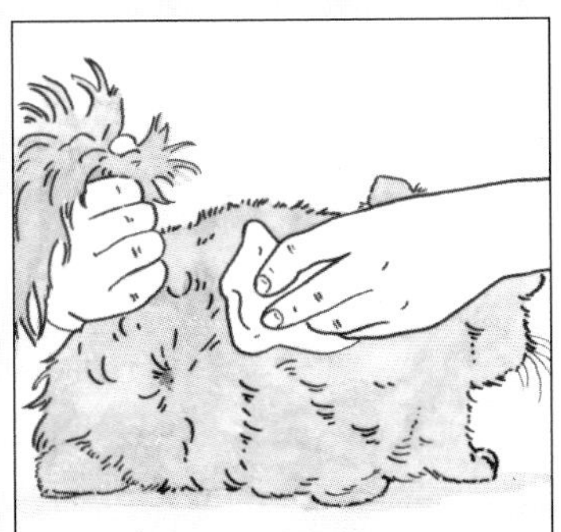

5) Clean a dirty anal region with a damp cloth.

Care of the Anus

If the cat's anus is sticky, wipe it clean with a damp cloth. A soiled anus is an indication of diarrhea (see page 85), which can have a great variety of causes, including errors in feeding, intestinal parasites, and infections. Persistent diarrhea in a cat is always the body's way of giving an alarm signal. Consult your veterinarian.

Nail Care

A cat that roams freely outdoors takes care of its own nails. It scratches them on trees (see photo, page 29). Indoor cats need a scratching post for that purpose (see page 10). Many cats, however, are quite disinclined to scratch. The nails on their front paws have to be cut several times a year with special clippers (available in pet stores). When using pet-nail clippers, make sure you remove only the tip of the nail, where no blood vessels are present. Watch the veterinarian a few times before you attempt the procedure yourself.

Proper Nutrition

Feral cats subsist for the most part on small rodents. Cats capture primarily mice and animals ranging up to the size of a rat. To a lesser extent cats also catch small birds and occasionally dine on insects and plant parts. Cats, according to some observers, devour their prey to the last morsel. In this way cats also obtain vegetable and mineral substances, which are present in the gastrointestinal tract of cats' prey. Some authorities, however, disagree that cats devour their prey to the last morsel.

Domestic cats that have adapted to living in the wild, as a rule, also subsist on the prey they hunt down, as well as on garbage that they find here and there. That usually is enough to satisfy their nutritional requirements.

Domestic cats that are allowed to roam freely persist in catching mice, even if those cats are fed regularly. It is not hunger alone, but also their characteristic hunting instinct, that induces cats to catch mice. Often the captured mouse is not even eaten, but is placed at the front door as a gift.

Although small prey is the cat's natural food, characteristic to the species, such prey is a great source of danger to the cat's health. Small animals are often carriers of pathogens and parasites that can infect your cat (see "Disorders Caused by Parasites," page 96, and "Infectious Diseases," page 104).

Hint: In "How-To: A Healthy Diet," page 18, we tell you how to feed your cat properly.

The Cat's Eating Behavior

The cat's behavior when eating is interesting. When you feed your pet, from time to time you may catch a glimpse of its natural behavior when hunting small prey.

Mice, as well as larger pieces of meat, frequently are not consumed right away, even if the cat is very hungry. A cat shakes its "prey," pulls chunks of meat off the dish, drags them around, and tosses them into the air. Sometimes it also hides them or swallows and regurgitates them. Even tiny kittens defend their "prey," growling and spitting at their brothers and sisters. If the food is mushy or liquid, however, several cats will lick or lap it from a bowl together without showing any possessiveness toward the food.

Feeding Times

By nature cats are accustomed to irregular feeding times. On occasion they can even go without food for a relatively long period, then devour huge quantities again. Your pet, however, should become accustomed to regular feeding times and standard amounts. That is the only way to check whether your pet has a healthy appetite or is rejecting his food because he doesn't feel well.

Outdoor cats, too, quickly get used to fixed feeding times. At these times you can maintain contact with outdoor cats and check on the state of their health.

You need to feed a young cat two to four times a day, an adult cat one or two times a day.

Hint: The food always has to be fresh and at room temperature. Never reuse leftover food: it is better to dispose of it and reduce the cat's portion the next time.

Food Amounts

Over time you will find out how much food your cat needs. If the cat is healthy and lively and maintains its approximate normal weight, its diet is adequate. It is best to use the serving sizes recommended on the commercial cat food packaging as a guideline, though these portions are often too large! Ask your veterinarian for advice regarding serving size based on your cat's metabolic rate and body condition.

Hint: Young cats and pregnant or nursing queens have greater nutritional requirements. For further information, please see "The Love Life of Cats," page 36. Old cats often eat less food (see "Tips on Feeding," page 44).

Drinking Is Important

The proper drink for a cat is water, which is the most important nutrient required to sustain normal cell function. Mammals can lose nearly all their reserves

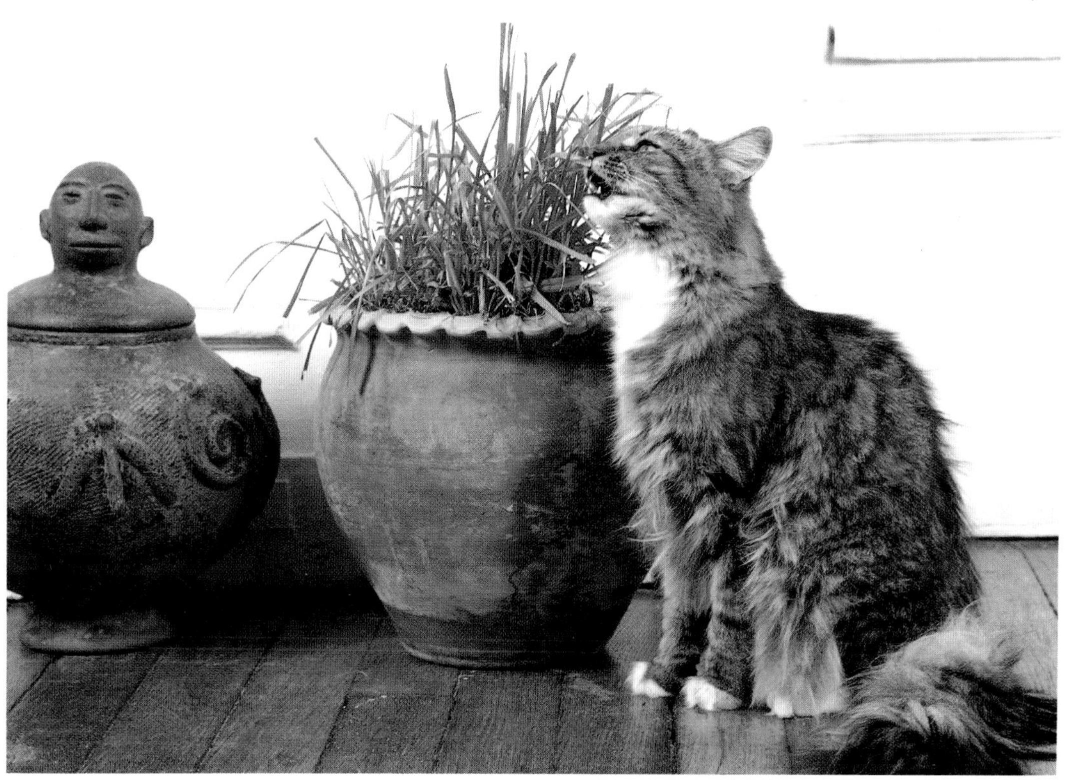

Most cats like to eat fresh greenery. It helps their digestion.

of glycogen and fat, half their protein stores, and 40 percent of their body weight and still survive. The cat, composed of nearly 70 percent water, is in severe metabolic disarray if it loses 10 percent of its body water. Death results if water loss rises to 15 percent. Fortunately, cats can concentrate their urine and conserve water. Nevertheless, your cat needs access to fresh, clear water at all times.

A cat that eats dry cat food needs to drink large quantities. For that reason it is best to soften the dry food in water before you serve the food to the cat.

Many cats prefer water that has been standing—in puddles, aquariums, and flower vases. These, however, are potential sources of bacteria. There are also cats that love to catch the drops of water from an open faucet.

The cat lapping milk is a long-familiar picture that is still a common sight in the countryside. Milk is a food of high nutritive value. Besides protein, it contains valuable minerals, especially magnesium and calcium. For nursing queens in particular milk is an important nutrient. Unfortunately, milk causes diarrhea in many cats because they cannot digest the sugar (lactose) contained in the milk. If your cat tolerates milk, it is all right for him to drink it. If he develops diarrhea, however, don't give him milk to drink under any circumstances.

HOW-TO: A Healthy Diet

As a result of scientific research, we know quite a lot about the nutritional requirements of cats. Consequently, many brands of commercial cat food contain everything of importance to cats' health. If, nevertheless, you would like to feed your pet homemade meals, you need to make sure that certain nutrients are present in sufficient quantities (see "Nutritional Disorders," page 20).

Commercial Cat Food

Commercial cat food is available in three varieties: dry, semimoist, and canned. Dry food is less expensive, easier to store, and more convenient to use than is canned food. Canned food is generally more palatable and, because it is three quarters moisture, is a better source of water than are other foods. (Dry food contains roughly 10 percent water. Semimoist has 33 percent.)

All three types of food can provide complete and balanced nutrition for your cat. To be sure you are buying a complete and balanced food, look for the following manufacturer's statement (or one synonymous with it) on the label: "[Name of food] provides complete and balanced nutrition for all stages of a cat's life as verified by feeding trials conducted in accordance with protocols established by the Association of American Feed Control Officials [AAFCO]."

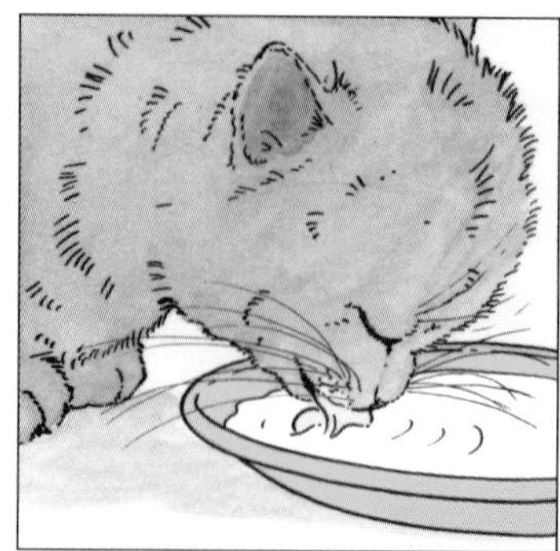

1) The cat curls its tongue as it drinks.

Some manufacturers' claims state that the food in question "has been formulated to meet the nutrient levels established in AAFCO's nutrient profiles." Because the nutritional performance of these foods has not been tested in feeding trials, you cannot be as certain of the foods' nutritional value as you can of a food evaluated on the basis of performance rather than formulation. You are safer, therefore, to buy foods that have been tested in feeding trials. (If you serve dry food, of course, the cat has to drink considerably more water than if you use canned food.)

Drinking

When a cat drinks, it curls its tongue downward and back, scooping the liquid into its mouth. Water is the natural drink for cats, not milk (see page 17).

Begging for Food

By living with cats, cat owners quickly learn to interpret their pets' various modes of behavior correctly. If a cat rubs against its human's legs, that often means "I'm hungry."

Home-prepared Food

Cats need a lot of high-grade protein—as a rule, animal protein. For that reason cat food has to have more protein than does dog food. Sources of high-quality protein—particularly muscle meats, organ meats, dairy products, and eggs—make a suitable basis for the diet.

Muscle meat and organ meat from horses, cows, rabbits, chickens, and turkeys represent the major source of protein in a cat's diet.

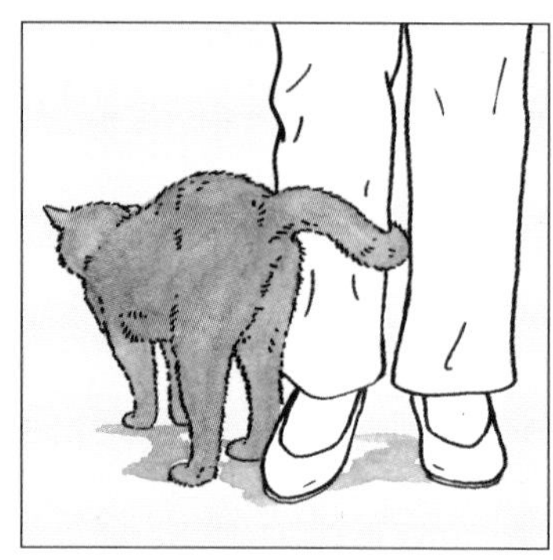

2) A cat owner knows: This cat wants food.

Important: All parts should be cooked before being fed to your cat.

Liver is an important source of energy and vitamins (especially Vitamin A). When raw it has a laxative effect, but in cooked form it can cause constipation. If a cat is fed liver exclusively or too frequently, however, it can develop Vitamin A poisoning (see page 71).

Fish, such as fillet of redfish or cod, is something that many cats enjoy from time to time. The fish should be served steamed and boned. One fish day per week is enough; otherwise, the cat's breath will have an overly fishy smell.

Cereal and vegetable products, including rolled oats, barley, rice, noodles, potatoes, and some vegetables—all in cooked form—can be given to your cat occasionally, in amounts of about three quarters to 1 ounce (20–30 g) per day. To keep the cat from "fishing out" the pieces of meat from its dinner, try pureeing the meal.

Vitamin-enriched margarine, offered now and then on your fingertip, is well received by cats, and it aids their digestion.

A raw egg yolk two or three times a week will ensure a beautiful, glossy coat of fur.

Bones are well suited for supplying the cat's body with minerals, but generally bones can be fed to cats only in the form of bone meal (please note the recommended amounts on the package). Don't give your pet poultry bones. They splinter easily and can get stuck in the cat's mouth (see "Problems Caused by Foreign Bodies" page 84).

Hint: Always enrich home-prepared food with a vitamin and mineral supplement (available from a veterinarian or in a pet store) to ensure that the cat is getting all the substances it requires (see "Nutritional Disorders," page 20).

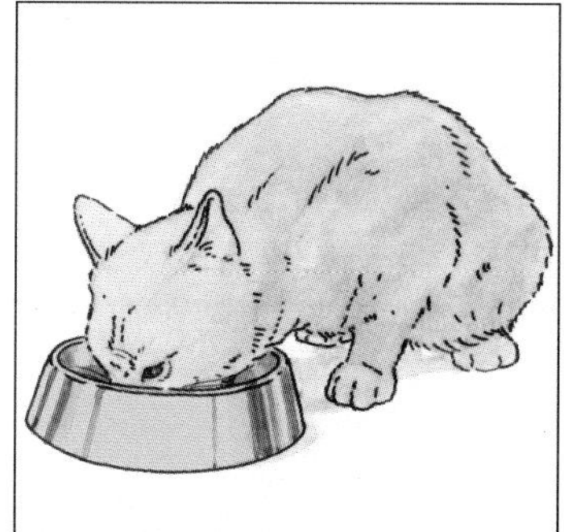

3) Cats often assume this crouching position next to their food bowl.

Tidbits from the Dinner Table?

If you live in close contact with your cat, you surely can't resist the temptation to give your pet a bite of your meal on occasion. Basically there is no reason not to—provided it is the exception rather than the rule. Make sure, however, that the food is not too heavily seasoned or sweetened (see "Nutritional Disorders," page 20).

Crouching over the Bowl

When they eat from their bowls, cats frequently assume a crouching position. Their front and rear legs are bent, and their hindquarters are slightly raised, while their tails are curled around their bodies.

Cat Grass

Most cats enjoy nibbling on fresh greenery and then regurgitating it immediately. Along with the plant parts, the cat brings up hair that it swallowed while grooming its coat and that has collected in its stomach. If you want to offer your housebound cat a special treat, give it some freshly sprouted grain, papyrus, or "cat grass," available in pet stores. Generally that will also keep your pet from nibbling on house plants (see pages 10 and 54).

Hint: Cats with long hair especially need fresh greens.

Avoiding Errors in Feeding

1. Cats are only too glad to let you make fussy eaters of them. A one-sided diet, however, will make your pet ill, so you need to watch nutritional balance.
2. Commercial dog food does cost less than cat food, but dog food contains too little protein. A cat would develop symptoms of nutritional deficiency from eating dog food (see page 21).
3. If you have several cats, each needs its own bowl so they all get plenty to eat.
4. After every meal clean the food bowls with hot water.

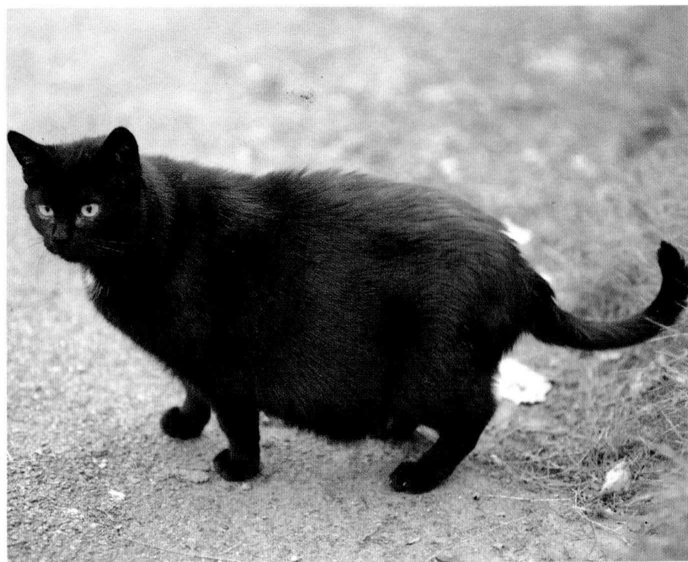
This cat is either pregnant, obese, or ill.

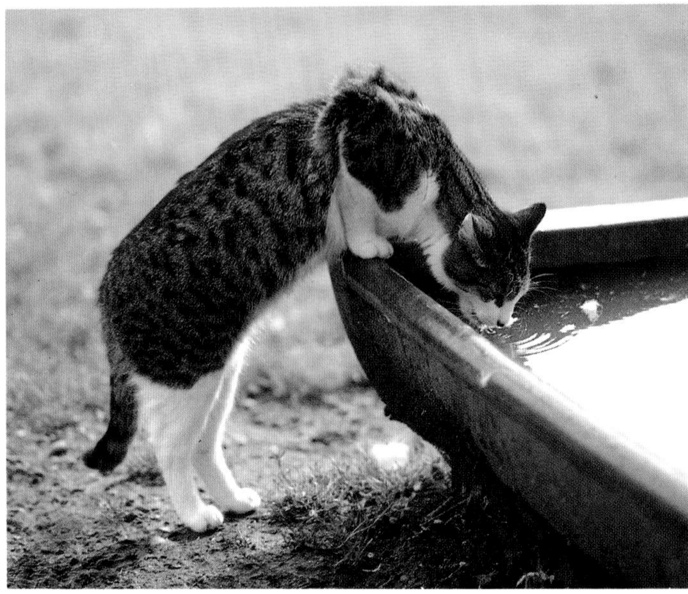
Feral cats rarely find enough to eat.

Nutritional Disorders

Serious illness can result if your cat gets too much or too little to eat, has an unbalanced, one-sided diet, or consumes spoiled or germ-infected food.

Fat Cats

An average weight of 5.5 pounds (2.5 kg) is normal for dainty purebreds like the Siamese, for example, while large-framed, powerfully built domestic cats weigh about 12 pounds (5.5 kg) on the average.

Moderate overweight is not detrimental to a cat's well-being, nor does a little extra weight shorten the animal's life expectancy.

Extreme overweight, however, places enormous stress on the cat's body. A potbelly is a telltale sign of obesity in cats. Cats that are too fat frequently have mobility problems as well. In addition, they become lethargic, and diseases of the liver, cardiovascular system, and joints can appear.

Too much fat, as a rule, is a problem only for indoor cats, who become obese usually as a result of being given too much food. A feral cat, however, that is dependent on catching its own food can never become too fat. In isolated cases indoor cats sometimes seem to suffer from a really excessive appetite. Their behavior becomes insistent, they constantly beg for food, and they swipe everything edible that they can get their paws on. A behavioral disorder probably is at the root of the voracious appetite.

In very rare cases, however, obesity can be caused by a pathological metabolic disorder or by a medication that has been administered.

Starvation diets are not tolerated well by cats and can lead to serious problems. If obesity has no pathological cause, first try cutting back slightly on your pet's rations. There are also low-calorie diet foods available, and they can be helpful in many cases (see "Special Diets," page 22). Weigh your cat periodically to see whether the diet is succeeding.

Giving your pet appropriate, balanced foods will prevent obesity. Tidbits from the dinner table and little treats to spoil your pet should be given infrequently.

Cats That Are Skin and Bones

Feral cats, in particular, that have no one to care for them become emaciated because they find too little food, and what they do find is not balanced. If well-cared-for house pets suddenly lose a great deal of weight, however, disease is the cause.

Emaciation is a symptom of almost all chronic organic and tumorous diseases. Infectious diseases also lead frequently to weight loss from lack of appetite. One possible cause is severe infestation by parasites, particularly gastrointestinal worms and tapeworms.

Uncastrated male cats lose a great deal of weight during rutting and roaming periods in particular, although no pathological disorder is present. Old cats also lose some weight.

Hint: If your cat's weight loss persists, it is essential to have the veterinarian discover the cause.

Malnutrition

A one-sided diet—for example, a predominantly vegetarian diet; a cat's preference for muscle meat, liver, or fish; or a diet consisting solely of home-prepared meals—can result in malnutrition. When that happens, the body of a cat lacks necessary substances such as certain amino acids, vitamins, and minerals; and this condition will lead to disease, even though the amount of food may be adequate.

Under- or oversupply of vital substances during a short period of time can be offset by the cat's system temporarily. Serious damage generally does not occur until the cat has been improperly fed for a relatively long span of time.

With home-prepared food it is virtually impossible to achieve the right balance for your cat. To do so requires a high level of expert knowledge and considerable expenditure as well. The most important substances that can cause ill health in your cat if they are lacking in its diet are:

- Vitamin B_1 (thiamine) deficiency can be caused by heating the cat's food (heat destroys the vitamin). The enzymes thiaminase in raw fish or avitine in raw egg white also destroy the vitamin. A deficiency can result in lack of appetite, weight loss, and nervous disorders in cats.
- Vitamin E deficiency occurs when the diet includes too much fish or meat. This deficiency results in lack of appetite and fatty-tissue disorders, including inflammations.
- Vitamin A deficiency can cause developmental disorders of the skeletal system, eye diseases, and fertility problems. A deficiency can result if no liver is used in home-prepared meals. With cats, however, an oversupply of Vitamin A is frequently of greater significance (see "Vitamin A Poisoning," page 71).
- Taurine is an aminosulfonic acid that is vitally important to cats. Taurine deficiency results from a predominantly vegetarian diet (cereal products, for example) or from eating commercial dog food. Taurine is especially crucial for pregnant and nursing queens; without it, young kittens have permanent damage (skeleton, nervous system). In adult cats taurine deficiency results in damage to the retina, impaired vision, blindness, and heart disease. By adding bottled clam juice (one teaspoonful daily) to home-prepared food, it is allegedly possible to prevent taurine deficiency.
- Arachidonic acid also has to be present in cats' food because cats cannot produce

this substance on their own. A deficiency, which is caused only by a one-sidedly vegetarian diet, can result in reproductive disorders and blood-clotting problems.

• Calcium deficiency can be caused by a diet of meat exclusively, as well as a diet in which cereal products predominate. It is primarily the calcium-phosphorus ratio in the food, which ideally is about 1:1, that is seriously disturbed in these diets. They contain a huge excess of phosphorus, which interferes with calcium resorption from the intestines. Calcium deficiency first becomes apparent in the blood. Hyperactivity of the parathyroid gland results, and that causes an increased amount of calcium to be drawn from the bones. This, in turn, can lead to motor disturbances and even to spontaneous fractures. Serious tooth damage can also occur.

Malnutrition can be avoided by using commercial cat food (see "How-to: A Healthy Diet," page 18). There is no objection to alternating commercial products with home-prepared meals for your cat.

Surplus of Vital Substances

An oversupply of some vital substances during a fairly long period of time also leads to pathological disorders that are equivalent to poisoning.

• A surplus of Vitamin A can be caused primarily by too much liver in a cat's diet. The locomotor system in particular suffers serious damage (see page 70). Vitamin A poisoning (see page 71) can also result from the use of too many vitamin supplements.

• A surplus of Vitamin D, in conjunction with an oversupply of calcium, leads to increased deposits of calcium, even outside the bone tissue. This can be prevented by feeding your pet commercial cat food, which has a balanced content of vitamins and minerals. If you feed your pet commercial cat food exclusively, there is no need to add special vitamin and mineral supplements, and their use could even be harmful.

Diseases Carried by Food

Prey and uncooked pieces of meat that may contain the infectious stages of gastrointestinal parasites, tapeworms, roundworms, other nematodes (see "Glossary," page 113), and the protozoan parasite *Toxoplasma gondii* can induce diseases, some of them serious, in cats (see "Disorders Caused by Parasites," page 96). Viruses and bacteria are also communicable to cats in this manner (see "Infectious Diseases," page 104). Raw pork can contain, among other things, viruses of Aujeszky's disease (see page 105), which is fatal to cats. Cooking, however, is a sure way to destroy all pathogenic organisms. Beef was thought to be a safe food for cats, but recently an infectious disease known as BSE or bovine spongiform encephalopathy (mad cow disease) has disconcerted many cat owners. The disease was first observed in English cattle. The pathogen attacks the cow's brain and causes BSE. Although transmission to cats is also possible, thus far it has not occurred to any significant extent.

Food Allergies

Under some circumstances various ingredients in commercially available cat foods can cause allergies (hypersensitivities) in cats. Frequently only a

Special Diets

In many cases specially formulated diets can allay or halt the progress of certain organic diseases and metabolic disorders.

Ready-to-serve diet foods are especially recommended. They are available from veterinarians.

Special diets are used primarily for overweight cats and cats with disorders like feline urological syndrome (see page 81), chronic renal insufficiency (see page 80), allergies (see page 77), and persistent diarrhea (see page 85).

There are also highly nutritious, protein-containing diet foods that can be given to your cat after a serious illness, for example, to get it on its feet again.

veterinarian is able to discern the connections.

Special diets (lamb with rice, for example) are helpful both in making the diagnosis (see "Allergies," page 80) and in alleviating the symptoms. When using such specially formulated diets, you need to make sure they contain all the essential nutrients.

Precautionary Measures

When a cat becomes a new member of your household, take the cat to a veterinarian as soon as possible. He or she will examine your pet thoroughly, verify that it has been vaccinated against the most dangerous infectious diseases (take along the vaccination record), determine what vaccinations may still be needed, and give advice about keeping a cat as a pet.

Controlling Parasites

Parasites like fleas, mites, and worms attack cats relatively frequently (see "Disorders Caused by Parasites," page 96).

External parasites such as fleas, ticks, and mites are treated—and killed—with gels, shampoos, or powders (available from veterinarians or pet stores).

Internal parasites such as roundworms, hookworms, and tapeworms can be detected in a stool test. Regular deworming treatments for your cat are important (see "Deworming Schedule," page 27).

Vaccinations

At the end of the eighteenth century, the English surgeon Edward Jenner discovered that cow milkers who became infected with cowpox (vaccinia) did not contract the fatal smallpox. On the basis of this finding, Jenner developed a vaccination procedure. He scratched the skin of healthy people to introduce the quite harmless cowpox pathogens, and in this way those people became immune to smallpox.

Times have changed since Jenner's day, and thus today's kittens are spared the aggravation of having a vile, repellant substance smeared into a scratch on their bodies. Yet the process initiated by the veterinarian's 22-gauge, stainless-steel needle is the same one that Jenner courted, and the object of the vaccine's pseudoinfection remains the same: the immune system, which begins to function at birth or shortly thereafter and which is one of the last of the body's systems to give up the ghost at death.

Newborn animals cannot produce antibodies efficiently because a newborn's lymphoid tissues do not operate at full strength. During gestation, kittens inherit immunity from their mothers—if their mothers have antibodies in their bloodstreams. Thereafter, kittens are protected by antibodies in their mothers' milk until the kittens are roughly eight weeks old.

For active protection by vaccination we utilize the body's

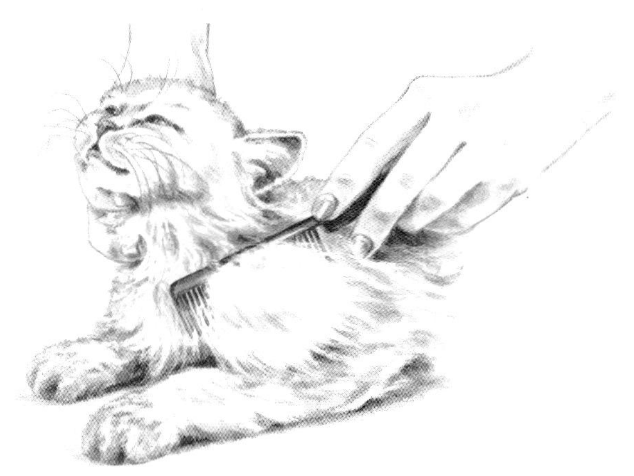

By combing your pet with a fine-toothed flea comb, you can tell whether the cat is infested with parasites like fleas and ticks.

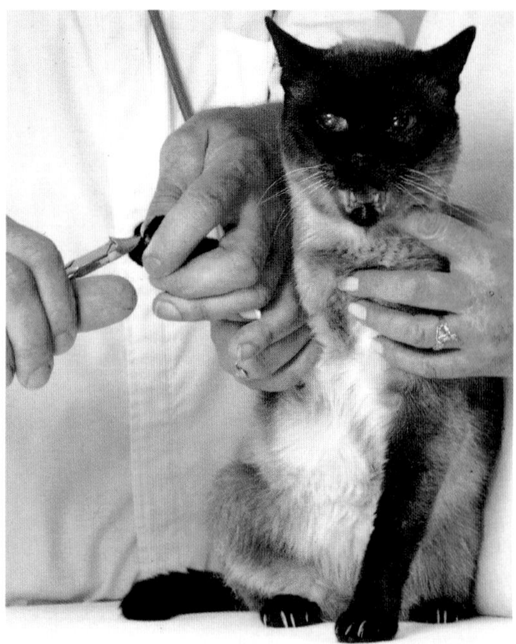

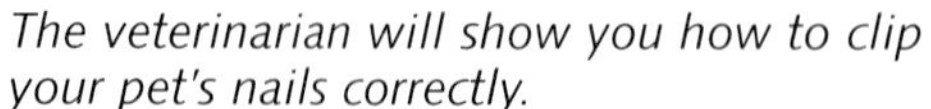

The veterinarian will show you how to clip your pet's nails correctly.

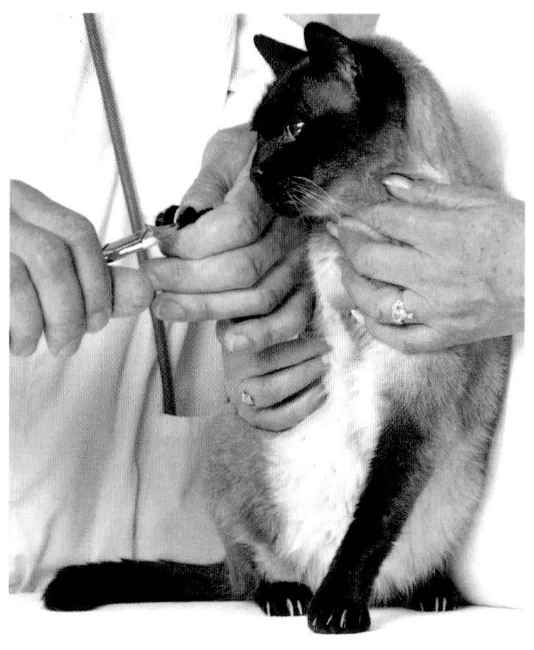

Be sure not to injure the blood vessels when you trim your cat's nails.

natural defense mechanism. If a pathogen (a virus or bacterium, for example) is implanted in the body, that virus acts as an antigen. That is, the animal vaccinated produces appropriate antibodies capable of fighting disease. This process takes at least one week. After that, the protective effect of an inoculation can last for a year or longer, depending on the vaccine.

Modern vaccines contain killed or living, modified pathogens. These cause an organism to produce specific antibodies, but they are, except in exceedingly rare cases involving modified-live vaccines, no longer capable of triggering a disease.

Vaccines exist that are effective against some of the most dangerous infectious diseases in cats. Responsible cat owners take advantage of the opportunity to safeguard their pets and themselves (see "Vaccination Schedule for Preventive Health Care," page 26).

Altering or Sterilization

Whether male or female, every cat that is not intended for breeding ought to be altered.

In *altering,* the reproductive glands (gonads) are surgically removed. In a male these are the testicles (castration); in a female, the ovaries (spaying). Through altering, the production of sex hormones, which takes place almost exclusively in the gonads, is prevented. Once the sex hormones are stopped, the sex drive is also extinguished. Neither male nor female cats suffer from the disappearance of their natural sex drive; on the contrary, altering has only a positive impact on the animal (see "Reasons for Altering," page 25).

In sterilization, the Fallopian tubes of the female or the seminal ducts of the male are severed or tied off. Production of sex hormones continues, and the sex drive remains intact. Only reproduction is rendered impossible. Sterilization is not appropriate for cats.

Hormonal Treatment

In queens used for breeding, estrus (see page 36) can be suppressed by treatment with certain hormones if no offspring are desired for the time being. Hormone therapy, however, has one drawback: It can promote diseases such as uterine infections (see page 82).

Hormone tablets are given to a female when estrus is to be suppressed for only a short time. Once the tablets are discontinued, the queen will go into heat again.

Hormone injections are administered when estrus is to be suppressed for a longer period of time (three to twelve months). Hormones also can be used to reduce the sex drive of potent males temporarily. Hormonal treatment is not recommended as a permanent solution; it is preferable to alter the animal.

Reasons for Altering

Altering is advisable for several reasons:

- It is a way to prevent uncontrolled reproduction among cats. In altered animals the sex drive is extinguished.

A female can bear her first litter when she is less than one year old. After a gestation period of two months, she gives birth to three to eight kittens and potentially can become pregnant again as soon as two weeks after delivery. This makes it immediately clear to what disastrous proportions the cat population can increase. Millions of domestic cats that have reverted to living in the wild will inevitably suffer unless humans intervene in the natural course of reproduction. If you have any notion of the way young and adult cats in many urban areas die a lingering death in a pitiful state (infections, starvation, accidents), you will realize that altering cats is of urgent concern to people interested in preventing cruelty to animals.

- With pet cats that are allowed outdoors the disappearance of the sex drive results in an increased tendency to stay close to home (on their owners' property). In general these cats behave with increased caution and are less apt to get into fights. There is an enormous decrease in the danger of infection through close contract with strange cats (sexual contact). Feral tom cats in particular develop a pronounced sex life. During rut they roam about for days and frequently change sex partners, often engaging in intercourse with cats that are ill. An unneutered male runs a much greater risk than does a neutered male of succumbing to an infection or dying in an

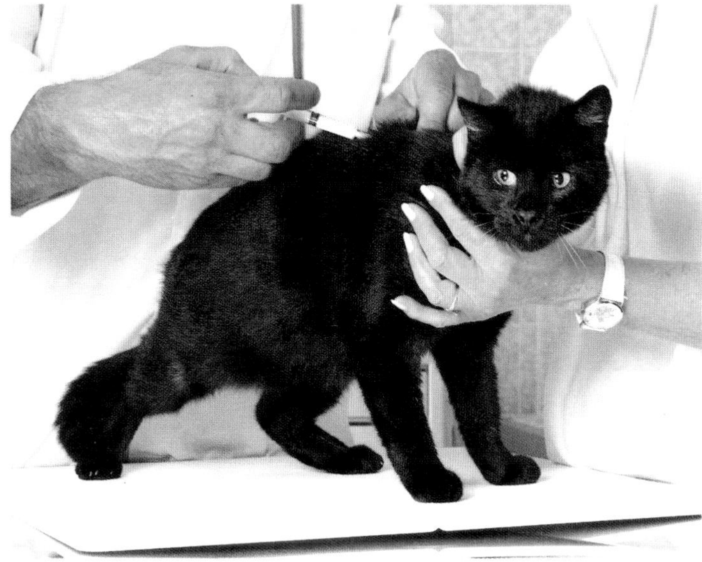

Vaccinations protect the cat against infectious diseases.

accident. He almost always looks pitiful, is emaciated and parasite ridden, and frequently is suffering with festering sores and debilitating injuries.

A neutered male, by contrast, usually is in top condition with a glossy coat and a well-balanced disposition. Neutered males and spayed females can live to the ripe old age of 20, often 10 times the life span of an unneutered cat.

Unspayed females in heat (see page 36) are affected by an incessant restlessness. They roll around on the floor, utter loud calls, and may spray urine around the house. This behavior can be an ordeal for cat owners' nerves. If the female never mates with a male during her estrus period, hormonal disorders sometimes result, and these can take the form of continuous or prolonged estrus (see page 36) and disorders of the ovaries and the uterus (see page 82).

Unneutered potent males generally cannot be kept indoors at all for any length of time. Few owners can tolerate their marking behavior, the spraying of urine (see page 34), which includes intense "qualities of fragrance."

The Process of Neutering

Males should be neutered at the onset of sexual maturity, which begins at roughly seven months of age. By that time sex-specific characteristics such as body proportions and head shape have developed fully. Neutering at an earlier time can allegedly result in urinary problems in male cats, though this remains unproven. Neutering is also possible in older animals, of course.

Cats that are allowed outdoors should be neutered in early spring before the main rutting season begins, if they are old enough.

Hint: Don't postpone neutering too long. If the male has already made extensive forays into the neighborhood during rut, he may retain this habit even after neutering.

Vaccination Schedule for Preventive Health Care

	Age	FPL	Feline respiratory disease	FeLV disease	Rabies	FIP
Basic immunization	8th week	•	•			
	12th week	•	•	•		
	16th week			•	•	•
	20th week					•
	after 1 year	•	•	•	•	•
	after 2 years	•	•	•	•	•
	after 3 years	•	•	•	•	•
	after 4 years	•	•	•	•	•

Important: Vaccinations are not effective immediately. It takes about one to two weeks for immunity to develop.

Female cats can be spayed quite early (at an age of six to twelve months) without harm, even before they reach puberty. Giving birth to at least one litter in her life is in no way essential to a female's development or her good health. On the contrary, the commonly occurring disorders of the ovaries and uterus are prevented by spaying. In our veterinary practice we have repeatedly observed kittens that went into heat at the tender age of six months and developed a uterine infection (see page 82).

Older females also can be spayed at any time. They frequently really begin to blossom and seem years younger.

Breeding queens that repeatedly have had problems giving birth are also candidates for spaying. Complications during labor may be congenital in origin. Spaying prevents the unfavorable genetic material from being passed on (see "Breed-related Problems," page 128).

The Surgical Procedure

Both females and males are operated on under general anesthesia. On the day before altering the animals should not be fed past 8:00 P.M. to avoid subjecting their circulation to unnecessary strain and especially to prevent complications caused by vomiting under anesthesia.

The surgical risk of altering is very low, thanks to modern operating techniques and anesthesia procedures. All veterinarians perform this routine operation in their offices. After surgery, the cat will probably be kept for observation at the veterinarian's office until at least the end of the day. Once home, the cat should remain indoors for at least seven to ten days.

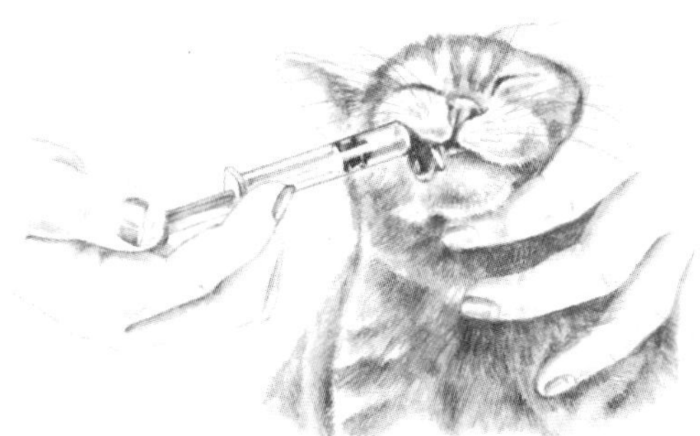

Liquid medications, administered with the help of a disposable syringe (without a needle), are introduced directly into the cat's mouth.

Deworming Schedule

Age	Timing	Interval
Young kitten	First treatment at 2 weeks of age	Weekly until the 12th week
Cats over 13 weeks old, adult cats	Every 3 months	
Breeding queens	14 days after delivery	Every 14 days until weaning
When severely infested with worms	Immediately	Repeat after 2–3 weeks

If microscopic examination of stool samples reveals that the worm infestation is no longer present and if the possibility of the cat's reinfection is slight, extremely frequent worm treatments are not necessary.

Typical Patterns of Behavior

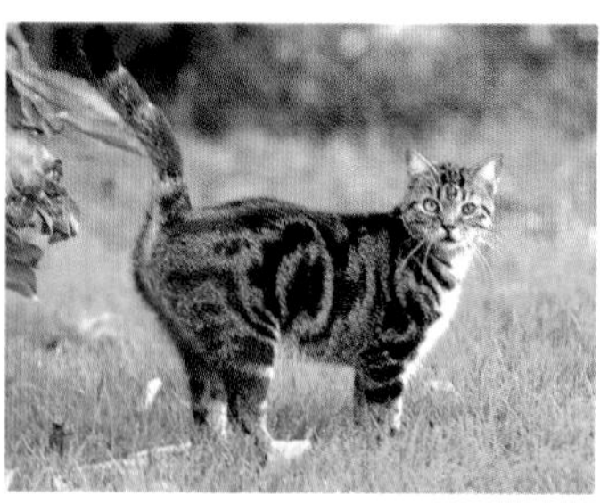

Cat owners who are well informed about the typical behavioral patterns of the feline species (in the photo above: a marking tom cat) can tell quickly whether their pets are healthy or ill. The first conspicuous symptoms of a disease in cats frequently take the form of altered modes of behavior.

Cats adore playing games. If your pet is not feeling well, it will lie listlessly on its bed or in some other private place.

The Typical Cat

Cats, like all other animal species, have characteristic patterns of behavior peculiar to their species. To understand these modes of behavior you first need to look at the wild original form of the cat. Down to the present day cats have retained many of their wild ancestors' behaviors, although modern cats have lived for centuries in close association with humans. Natural patterns of behavior are innate, and they are passed on to subsequent generations. For this reason, in certain situations cats have no choice but to react true to type rather than voluntarily.

By nature cats tend to be solitary animals. In their territories they rule alone and roam through them searching for prey. A cat seeks out other cats only for the purposes of mating and raising kittens.

Since the cat is a loner rather than a pack animal, it lets itself be subjugated to a human less readily than does a dog.

Cats that live in close association with humans, however, can develop strong bonds with those persons, bonds that often are stronger than the attachment to other cats. If a cat has only scant contact with a human, that person will be merely the dispenser of its food, whom the animal otherwise encounters with mistrust.

Hunting Behavior

The cat is a hunter whose natural quarries are primarily animals the size of a mouse, but may also include a lesser amount of small birds. The cat lies in wait for a mouse, creeps up on it without making a sound, and finally captures it, pouncing with lightning speed. The cat wraps its front paws around the mouse and kills it with a single bite to the back of the neck. To a certain extent this fatal bite seems to be a learned behavior. Cats that have not learned from their mothers how to kill a mouse are certainly able to catch a mouse later on but not to kill it properly. For wild cats that live in their natural surroundings, stalking and catching prey—behavior learned as they play—is essential to survival.

Humans can observe the decline of the stimulus threshold in pet cats that have little or no opportunity to develop their prey-catching drive fully. A cat, even when at play, will pay close attention and assume a stalking posture when reacting to a small, movable object such as a little ball or a piece of crumpled paper. Quickly removing the object evokes a dash or a pounce with attempts at capture. The cat's biting of the object, clutching it with its front paws, and working it over with its rear paws

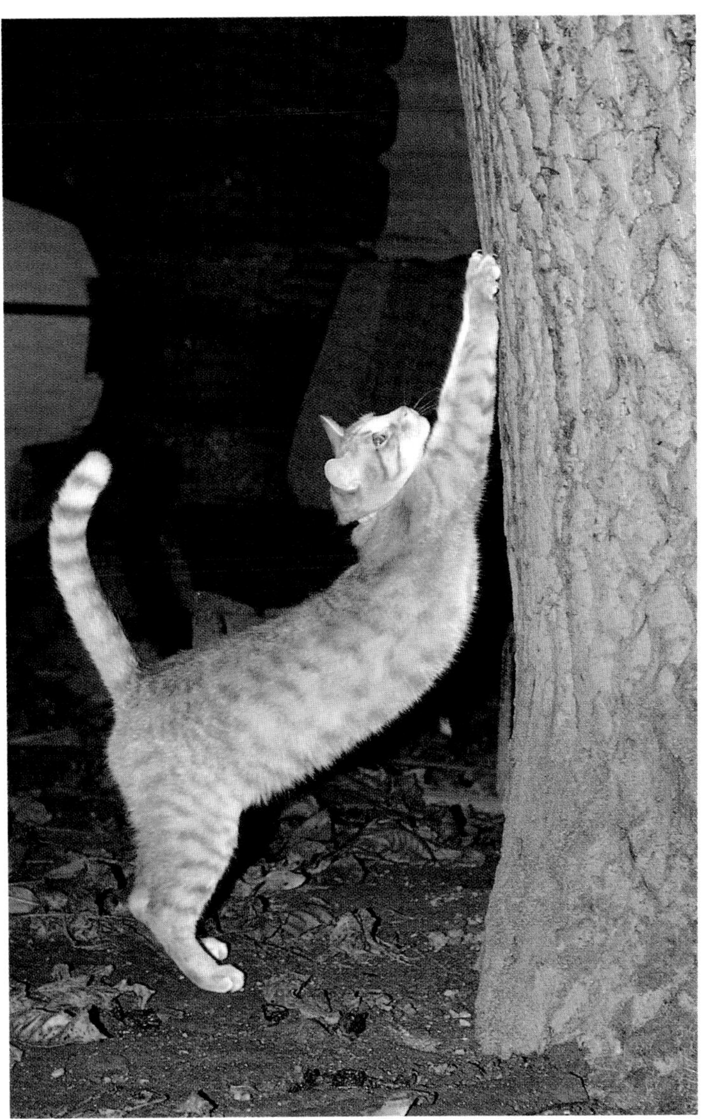
The cat removes the dead husks of its claws when it scratches on trees.

while lying on its side are all part of a coordinated effort to overpower a small quarry. The longer the cat is deprived of an opportunity to act out this prey-catching drive, the lower the stimulus threshold will drop. Finally, even the hand of its familiar owner, when moved quickly away from the cat, will be considered a substitute quarry.

Hint: Never use your bare hand as an object of play. It could get scratched (see "Scratches," page 47, and "Important Notes," page 127).

Taking Cover

The cat, unlike the dog, is not an untiring runner. For that reason, when fleeing from an unpleasant situation or a frightening object, a cat endeavors to find cover as quickly as possible and to remain there.

A human can sometimes take advantage of this behavior pattern when a cat has escaped in unfamiliar surroundings (at a cat show, when being taken to the veterinarian, or on vacation). If this happens, don't immediately take up pursuit; that would only cause the animal to continue to flee. Keep your eye on it until it stops running and remains in one place. Then approach the cat carefully, acting as if you don't notice it and intend to walk right past it. Once you are close enough, speak soothingly to the animal and, moving slowly, try to stroke it and, finally, to take hold of it.

Attack as an Anxiety Reaction

Feline attack behavior does not refer to the overpowering of prey. This term is applied instead to the cat's anxiety reaction in a situation where flight is impossible. The attack is heralded first by hissing. Not until the cat feels directly threatened does it rush forward and employ its claws and teeth in self-defense. In technical terminology we say that there is a critical distance short of which an animal will attack.

A human can trigger attack behavior in a cat by driving it into a corner, locking it in a cage, or holding it against its will. A mother cat that feels threatened but cannot run away because her strong bond to her young makes flight impossible will defend herself with her teeth and claws.

Aggression among cats also results from rivalries or territorial behavior (a strange cat enters another cat's territory). Then the cat's ears are laid back, its whiskers are spread wide, and its pupils are dilated, depending on the anxiety state. Its tail is lowered and bent in a hook shape, and its hair stands on end (see illustration, page 31). One cat crouches in front of the other, then leaps on top of it. The other cat parries with the speed of lightning, rolling over on its back (to keep the attacker from seizing its nape) and using its teeth and claws (see illustration, page 34).

When male cats fight, they first stare at each other, sometimes for minutes at a time. Only the tips of their tails quiver with excitement while they are thus engaged. Fights of this type sometimes end with bloody wounds caused by biting.

Play Behavior

The play instinct is extremely pronounced in cats. As they play, they practice all the vital patterns of behavior and explore the world around them.

A cat's mother and littermates are first of all its playmates. With them it experiments with social as well as fighting behaviors, patterns that later can be observed when the cat is engaged in rivalry or defending its territory and prey. Cats also use prey such as mice or rats for play, however. Humans are also accepted willingly as playmates. Many cats delight their owners with their exuberant play behavior well into old age.

Other Behaviors

Some modes of a cat's behavior toward humans are derived from its inborn grooming instinct, its natural behavior as a kitten toward its mother, and its sexual behavior. These unmistakably include:

- Licking, affectionate nibbling, and biting of the human hand.
- "Kneading" with the front paws.
- Purring when contented.
- Behavior of queens in heat toward humans.

Licking the hand: During the first few weeks of her kittens' lives, the mother cat licks their anal regions thoroughly with her tongue. This "massage" is the only way for the baby cats to pass stool and urine. A male cat licks kittens or a female he is courting as proof of affection.

"Kneading" or "treading" with the front paws: This behavior toward humans is traceable to the time when the cat was nursing. It pushed its forepaws against its mother's teats to stimulate the milk flow.

Purring: Very early, kittens nestled against their mother's side begin to proclaim their well-being by purring. In dealing with humans as well cats signal their contentment by purring. It should not be taken as proof of their good health, however; sick cats can also purr.

Insistent behavior: A cat in heat displays her natural sexual behavior to her familiar human as well. She rolls back and forth in front of her owner and turns her hindquarters toward him or her, raising her rear end when her back is gently stroked (see also page 36).

Body Language

Cat owners who pay close attention to their cats will soon be able to recognize their pets' moods from certain physical expressions. You will be able to interpret the cat's offering its head, putting its tail up into the air, cuddling up to your side, and licking as signs of friendly approach. You will also be able to classify these correctly: thumping its tail, assuming a crouching position with ears put back, hissing, and bristling its hair. If your cat is in such a mood, even as the result of playing, do not provoke it further.

Behavioral Problems

Problems naturally can arise in any close association between a cat and a human. Many of the cat's behavior patterns are annoying and unpleasant for cat owners, but they are in complete conformity with the natural modes of behavior of a healthy cat.

Abnormal patterns of behavior rarely appear in cats, and such behaviors frequently are attributable to errors made by humans in dealing with cats. Even less common is pathologically disturbed behavior.

Training a cat is far more difficult to accomplish than training a dog for example.

Desirable behaviors can be fostered with treats and words of praise, but your efforts will not cause the cat to react the way you want every time and in every situation in the future.

Undesirable behaviors can rarely be unlearned by cats. Punishment should be administered only with extreme caution, because a cat connects the punishment (for example, being yelled at or squirted with water) only with the punisher, not with the action that elicited the punishment. A friendly, affectionate kitten can quickly turn into a difficult, shy, or even aggressive cat. Where fights over differences of opinion are concerned, cats are downright unforgiving animals.

Conflict situations that arise when you live with a cat are discussed below. Only general suggestions on how to avoid or handle such situations can be given here. A veterinarian or a cat behavior specialist who is familiar with behavioral problems, however, often—after ruling out pathological causes—can determine the connections by talking with you. He or she may then work out some suggested solutions.

Problem: Shyness

The cat is timid and repeatedly hides under the furniture.

Possible causes:

- Genetic predisposition (has the nature of a wild animal).
- Change in environment (new apartment, for example).
- Insufficient attention from humans during the cat's development as a kitten.
- Improper behavior by humans (rigorous punishment, for example).

What you can do: If there is a genetic predisposition, only modest progress can be made. In most cases quite a lot is achieved by waiting and showing friendly attention. To build the necessary trust you can begin by repeatedly offering the cat small amounts of food from your hand. Under no circumstances should you treat the cat impatiently, catch it, or hold it tightly. Children, too, need to learn to respect the cat's special personality. The cat will decide when it is in the mood for contact.

Problem: Scratching and Biting

Although the cat is not shy, it is reluctant to let itself be touched. It scratches, bites, and throws itself on its back.

Possible causes:

- Improper handling of the young cat, often by young children.
- Prey-catching and fighting games in which the cat's owner uses his or her bare hands.

What you can do: If the cat scratches or bites during a wild play session, make its overly

Fur bristled, nails extended: This cat is about to strike.

rough behavior clear to it by simply stopping the game without punishment and going away. Sometimes the cat will also react to a human's loud moaning. Similar methods are applicable if the cat climbs up people's legs and clothing, using its claws to do so.

Hint: When playing games that involve catching, scratching, and biting, always use objects (small ball, cloth mouse, crumpled paper). Use your hands only to pet the cat in a relaxed atmosphere. Make sure that children behave accordingly.

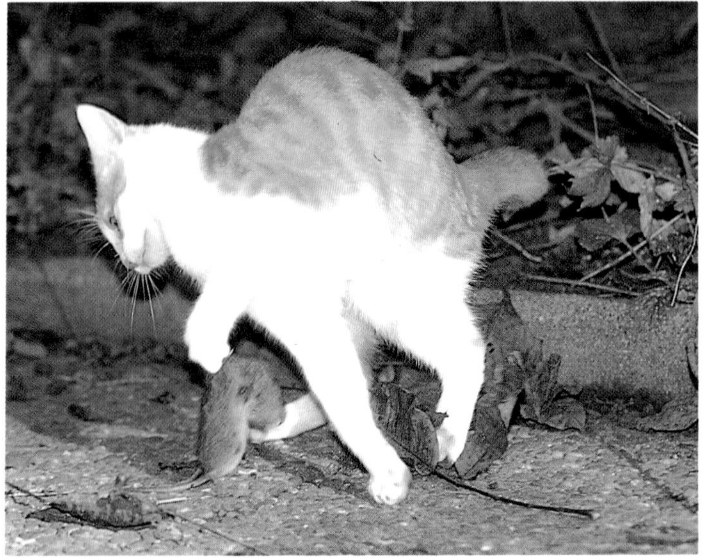

Over and over again the rat is tossed into the air.

Problem: Scratching Objects

The cat scratches furniture, wallpaper, and the like.

Possible cause: Natural behavior that is used to groom nails and mark territory.

What you can do: If you are unwilling to resign yourself to living in a home "decorated" by a cat try to:

• Keep the cat out of rooms with furniture and wallpaper that you don't want scratched under any circumstances. (Don't leave doors to off-limits rooms open!)

• Provide a scratching tree, scratching post, or scratching mat, and praise the cat every time it scratches there.

• Spray the cat with a water pistol every time it gets ready to scratch on a forbidden object. The cat should connect this unpleasant experience not with you but with her scratching on the object. In the future she will be less likely to scratch there.

Problem: Rejecting Food

The cat eats with very poor appetite or rejects the nutritionally balanced meal intended for it.

Possible cause: If a medical disorder can be ruled out, then improper feeding is commonly at the root of this problem.

• If your kittens are fed one food exclusively, later on they may want to eat only that food. They are fixated on its smell and taste.

• If you constantly feed a cat tidbits like beefsteak, calf's liver, sausage, or ham, you are taking the risk that the cat soon will refuse to eat anything else. This one-sided diet will result in medical problems (see "Nutritional Disorders," page 20).

• The cat can develop an aversion to a certain food if it connects eating with unpleasant experiences (for example, spoiled food or food mixed with bitter-tasting medications).

• Many cats lose their appetites if they are not fed by their humans from their customary bowls and in their usual places.

What you can do: Even kittens need to be accustomed to a variety of foods if at all possible, including commercial cat food in particular, which later on will be their main source of nourishment. Adult cats need only one serving of

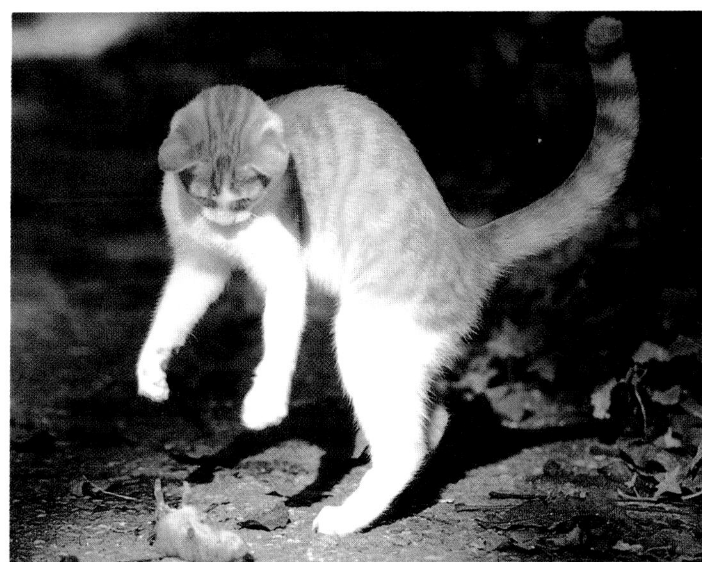

The cat satisfies its prey-catching instinct by playing with its prey.

food daily in order to stay healthy and keep from becoming overweight (see "Proper Nutrition," page 16). The food should be fresh and served at room temperature, and it should be well balanced.

If the cat no longer accepts such food with great enthusiasm, that is no reason to begin spoiling the animal immediately with choice morsels. If a cat eats only a certain food or delicacies, in the interest of the animal's health you need to get it used to normal commercial cat food. Let's use the example of liverwurst. First, offer the cat liverwurst mixed with a little canned cat food. Then gradually increase the proportion of cat food until your pet is eating canned food with only a trace of liverwurst and, finally, is eating unadulterated canned food alone.

Problem: Rivalry Among Cats

Your cat fights with another cat.

Possible causes: There are several possible reasons for this behavior.

- For cats, defending their territories against other cats is a natural mode of behavior, more pronounced in some cats than in others. Almost all cats lay claim to at least a small place reserved for themselves alone.
- When space is at a premium, aggression develops between sexually mature (unaltered) animals. Sexually mature tom cats in particular can never live together in close quarters because of their rivalry.
- It often happens that a mutual aversion suddenly arises between cats that have lived together peacefully for a long time. The dislike can be so intense that bitter fighting results. Animals with no chance to flee (indoor cats) thus run the risk of serious injury. Among feral cats one animal generally tries to switch to a new territory.

If a male cat feels a strong dislike for a female, he does not view her as a sexual partner even when she reaches the peak of estrus (see page 36). Instead, he attacks her vehemently. Even well-known researchers have no adequate explanation for such personal animosities between two cats.

What you can do: There are a few things you can try.

- If you would like to acquire a second cat as a companion for your pet of long standing, choose a young kitten if possible. Young animals are more likely to be tolerated and treated with less aggression than are mature cats. Usually young cats are accepted after a brief acclimation period.

Nonetheless, at first you should use a wire barrier (or a cage) to protect even little kittens from the attacks of established cats. If the new cat is an adult, such safeguards are absolutely essential. The cats can see, smell, and hear each other, and they are able to make initial contacts without danger. If you have the impression that they like or at least tolerate each other after an adjustment period of several days, then you can risk leaving the cats in a room together under supervision.

If you want to start out with two pet cats, it is advisable to acquire two kittens at the same time. In general, it is true that the more room you can offer the cats for living and keeping out of each other's way, the less likely they are to engage in aggressive behavior.

• Animals that are not being kept for breeding purposes should be altered at the proper time.

• There definitely are some cats that can never live together and that you can never bring to accept each other, despite patient effort. If your cats fall into this category, you have to either keep them separated or give one of them away.

Problem: Soiling in the House

The cat refuses to use the litter box or sprays urine onto the walls.

Possible causes:

• This may be marking behavior, which is developed especially by sexually mature male cats. You can recognize marking with urine (spraying) this way: The cat will raise its hindquarters and tail into the air and, trembling, spray a stream of urine onto objects. For sexually mature tom cats in particular, defecating in certain places also seems to have a marking function.

• The sudden onset of soiling that is not attributable to marking behavior can be caused by an illness (for example, an intestinal or urinary tract infection, discussed on page 80).

• The cat's box is located in the wrong place (right next to the food bowl, for example); the litter doesn't appeal to the cat; the litter box is not emptied or cleaned often enough; the smell of disinfectants has spoiled the litter box for the cat.

• Serious changes in the environment can also lead to soiling by cats: moving to a new home; sudden restriction on entering certain areas of the house; new furnishings. The intrusion of new cohabitants (a cat, a dog, a human) into a cat's area or the appearance of tensions in a household with several cats can also disturb the animal's emotional balance.

What you can do: Your course of action will depend on the cause.

• Where marking behavior is concerned—particularly spraying by sexually mature males—altering almost always is a speedy, permanent remedy (see page 24), unless the behavior is long term, in which case other methods of treatment will be needed in addition.

• If a pathological disorder is present, only a veterinarian can help.

• All other types of soiling place great demands on the empathy and psychological understanding of the cat owner and the veterinarian.

First, the cat's litter box has to be made appealing. Fill it with a litter that the cat accepts. The litter has to be cleaned or even changed daily, and for some cats several cleanings are necessary each day. Some cats prefer uncovered litter boxes, but most will readily accept cave-like structures.

If you have done everything listed above and your cat still

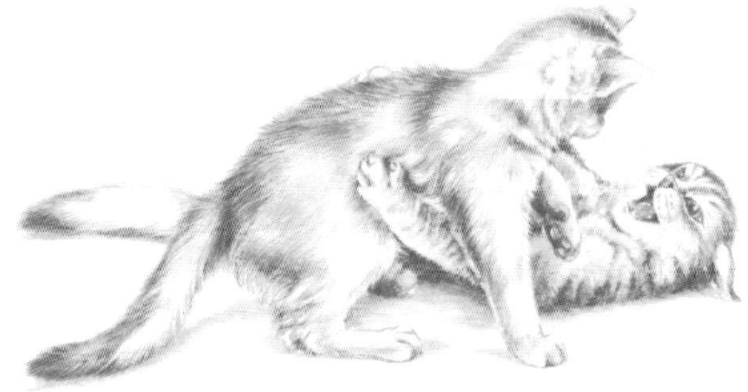

Young kittens practice fighting behavior as they play.

persists in defecating or urinating in one or more places in your home, you can try the following: Put litter boxes at the spots your pet favors, and get it accustomed to using them there; change the floor covering; set up the cat's food and water bowls there.

- In general, there is the possibility of using counter-conditioning to keep the cat away from certain places where it does undesirable things. If you catch your pet in the act, spray it with a squirt gun or water bottle.
- If the cat prefers a certain kind of undersurface for its "business"—such as newspapers, bed sheets, or pieces of carpeting—it is possible to lay this material in the cat's box and gradually replace it with standard litter.
- If the cat first is locked in a small room with a smooth floor surface (a bathroom, for example), it usually will accept a litter box set up there as its only alternative, unless the cat has developed a preference for smooth floors. Once your pet is using the litter box, you can experiment with letting the cat out into larger areas of your home. If you want the litter box to stand permanently in a certain place, it will have to be shifted there gradually.
- If all efforts fail in your cat's case, all that remains is the possibility of getting your pet used to going outside or giving it away to someone who will keep it as an outdoor cat.

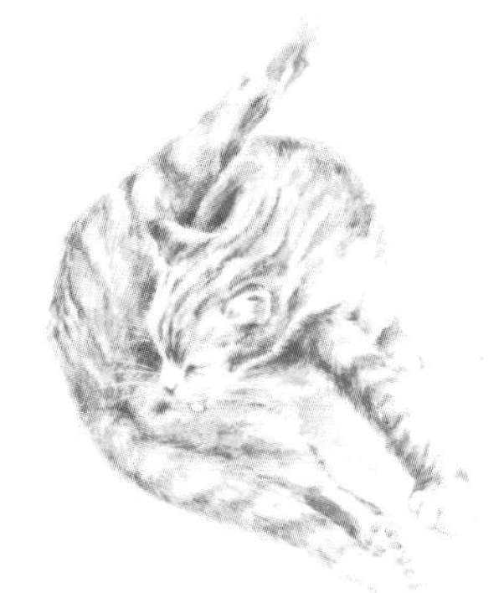

Cats are very clean animals by nature.

Behavior Counseling

If a medical problem has been treated or ruled out and your cat's unfortunate behavior persists, you can seek help from a behavioral consultant. You must be careful if you do, however. All cat behaviorists are not created equal. They vary immensely in training, background, and experience. If you do not choose wisely, you could spend a lot of money and still have a cat that soils the carpet all the time.

The persons best qualified to cope with problem animals are certified applied animal behaviorists. These individuals have met the educational, experiential, and ethical standards set forth by the Animal Behavior Society—the largest scholarly organization in North America devoted to the study and understanding of animal behavior (see "Information," page 126). A certified applied animal behaviorist must have a graduate degree in animal behavior, must have demonstrated expertise in using behavioral principles, and must have supervised consulting experience.

Number Please

The telephone numbers of local, regional, and national animal hotlines are available from veterinary associations and animal shelters. The qualifications and the level of expertise of the persons on the other ends of those hotlines are quite varied. A few hotlines are staffed by well-qualified experts. Other hotlines are handled by volunteers whose training and supervision range from extensive to minimal. Still other hotlines play back prerecorded audiotapes that provide general information.

Brief conversations or tape-recorded messages do not afford the opportunity to analyze individual cases thoroughly. At the very least that requires a telephone call of twenty minutes or more. For complicated or longstanding problems such as aggression, a phone call may not be adequate. An in-home visit by a behaviorist and several followups are probably necessary.

The Love Life of Cats

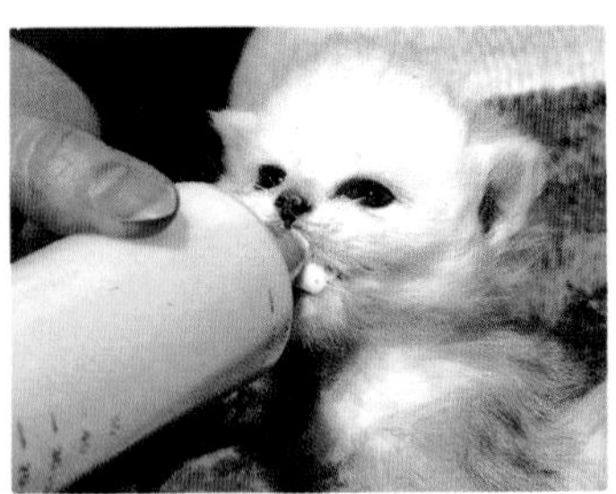

The sight of young kittens causes many a cat fancier's heart to leap with joy. There is wild tussling over the mother cat's teats as the little kittens try to push each other away from the sought-after milk source with their tiny paws. If a cat has more than six babies, it may be that some of them are getting inadequate nourishment or even no nourishment at all. You can rear such little cats with a special pet nurser.

Heat in Females

The female cat's period of sexual excitement is known as heat, or estrus. At the onset of puberty—between the sixth and twelfth months of life—the cat comes into heat for the first time. She seems restless, utters calls, rolls around, and presses herself to the ground. Free-roaming cats rove around. Indoor cats, however, pay court to familiar humans. Cats stretch their hindquarters into the air when you stroke their backs, and they tread up and down with their hind legs as soon as you touch their rear thighs.

An unspayed female (see "Altering or Sterilization," page 24) comes into heat two or three times a year for about nine days at a time. If no mating takes place, she sometimes can remain in a state of sexual excitement for two to three weeks. If the cat goes a fairly long time without mating, hormonal disorders can result. They easily can develop into an infection of the uterus (see page 82).

Continuous or Prolonged Heat

If an indoor cat does not mate during the approximately one-week heat phase (this virtually never occurs in free-roaming cats), the period of sexual receptivity will recur in a three-week cycle. If the cat continues to come into heat without mating, the heat can become so prolonged that the boundaries between the individual cycles are no longer evident. This state, known as continuous or prolonged heat, usually is accompanied by the formation of ovarian cysts.

Mating Readiness in Males

In contrast to the queen, a healthy, sexually mature tom is ready to mate at any time. He is not choosy in regard to his sex partner—apart from mutual antipathies between the two, of course. The male often demonstrates his readiness to mate by spraying: His tail quivering, he sprays objects with his urine. By wailing, licking his penis, and running restlessly back and forth in front of his adored one, he shows her that he is in the mood for romance.

The Stud Cat

If you want to breed your purebred queen, don't use just any male as a stud; make a concerted effort to find a suitable male. Attend a cat show or ask breeders for information. Breeders will be able to tell you what you need to take note of (for example, the requisite vaccinations and the stud fees).

The Act of Mating

Although a queen at the peak of estrus usually

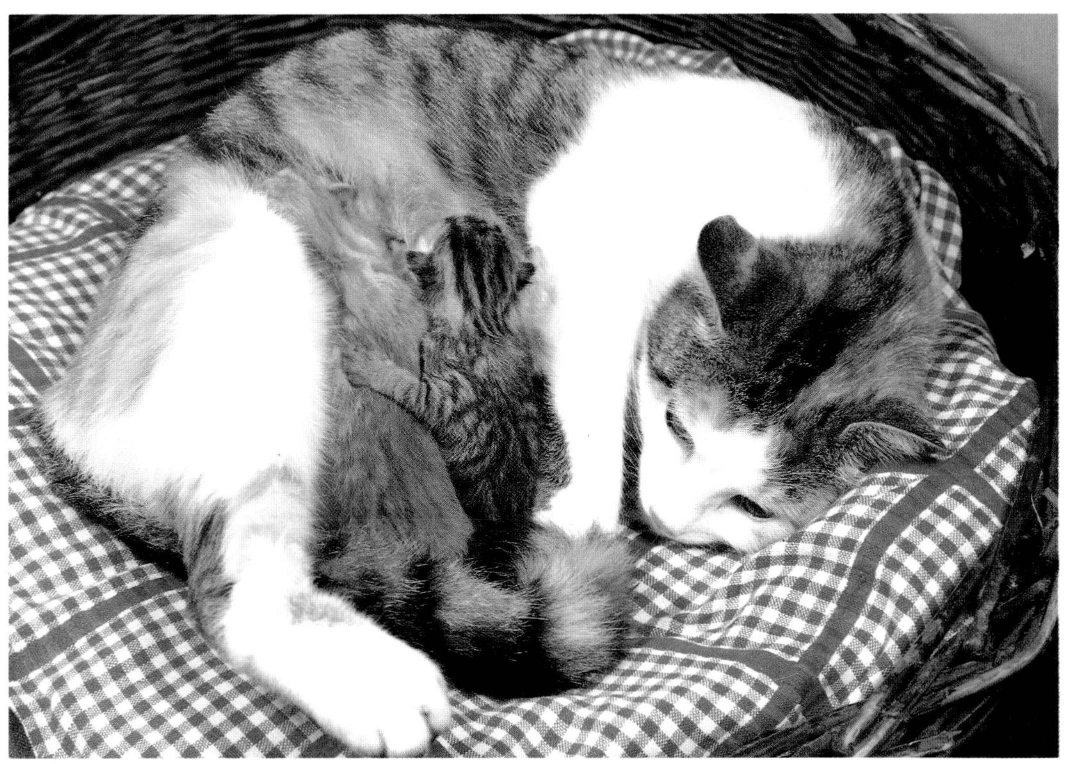

The kittens stimulate the flow of breast milk by pushing against or "kneading" their mother's abdomen with their forepaws.

announces her willingness to mate to a love-hungry tom in no uncertain terms, he may be standoffish at first. Only after fairly lengthy mutual courting and meowing does he suddenly make an attempt. He mounts the female from behind and seizes the nape of her neck in his teeth (see illustration, page 38). The act of mating is possible only if the female actively participates. If, after some effort, the male succeeds in inserting his penis and ejaculating, she emits a loud cry. After mating is completed, the male takes to his heels in a swift bound because the hissing female usually gives him a cuff with her paw. She rolls vigorously several times and licks her genitals, while he, at a safe distance, waits for a renewed opportunity. Usually they mate more than once.

Pregnancy

If the mating was fertile—that is, if the female has conceived—she will not go into heat again except in very rare instances.

Signs of pregnancy: From the third week on you can tell a cat is pregnant by the change

HOW-TO: Kittening

Mating Behavior

If the female is willing to mate, she crouches down, elevates her hindquarters, moves her tail to one side, and treads up and down with her hind legs. Now the male can mount her, taking hold of her coat at the nape of her neck, and inserting his penis into her vagina. Following ejaculation, the male's withdrawal is usually accompanied by a piercing cry from the female.

Fertility and Gestation

In contrast to many other animal species that ovulate spontaneously, the cat ovulates in response to the act of mating. The egg cell, or ovum, which is released between 25 and 36 hours after mating, travels through the Fallopian tube toward the uterus. Eggs can be fertilized there only during a brief period of time. The male's sperm, too, has limited viability. Within 48 to 72 hours the spermatozoa have to unite with an ovum that is capable of being fertilized.

You can figure out the probable delivery date on your own (63 days after the first mating occurs). Variations of six days are normal. After 10 days of gestation, the embryo already is 10 millimeters long. The fetus grows about 3 millimeters per day—more slowly at the beginning and more rapidly toward the end of the term—reaching a length of about 5 inches (13 cm) by the day of delivery.

The Kittening Box

As the time of delivery approaches, the cat becomes restless and looks for a suitable kittening place. A cat that is very used to human company will become visibly more relaxed if she can give birth in a prepared kittening box under constant supervision.

Equipment: Most suitable is a cardboard box lined with a thick layer of newspaper on which clean sheets are placed. The kittening box should measure about 24 × 16 inches (60 × 40 cm) with a height of 14 inches (35 cm). At one end cut a low entrance near ground level. Cover one half of the box with a lid.

Location: Put the kittening box in a quiet place that is warm and free from drafts.

After the birth: Remove the damp newspaper and put clean sheets in the kittening box.

Litter box for the young: As soon as the little kittens can leave the kittening box on their own, you need to set up a shallow litter box for their use. A plastic pan about 2 inches (5 cm) high, 20 inches (50 cm) wide, and 24 inches (60 cm) long filled with cat litter, is very suitable for that purpose.

Raising the Baby Cats

Normally the raising of the young in the first few weeks is unproblematic. The queen handles everything on her own.

You need to feed the nursing queen three or four times a day. She needs about 16 ounces (450 g) of nutritionally complete (canned) cat food per day. In addition, you can give her a restorative preparation (available from your veterinarian or in pet stores) that contains proteins, minerals, vitamins, and trace elements.

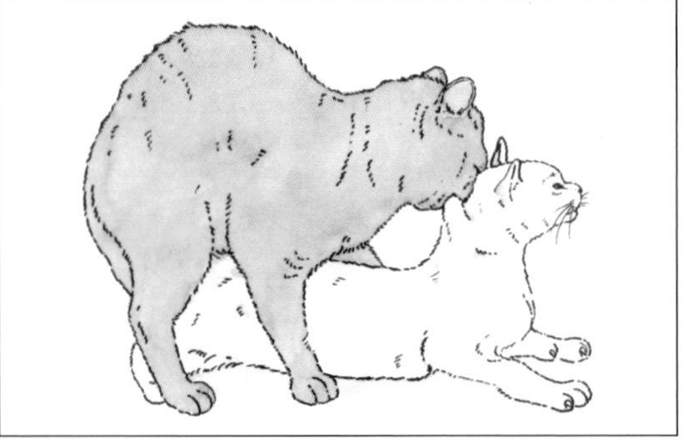

1) Cats in the act of mating: Several infectious diseases and external parasites can be transmitted when cats mate.

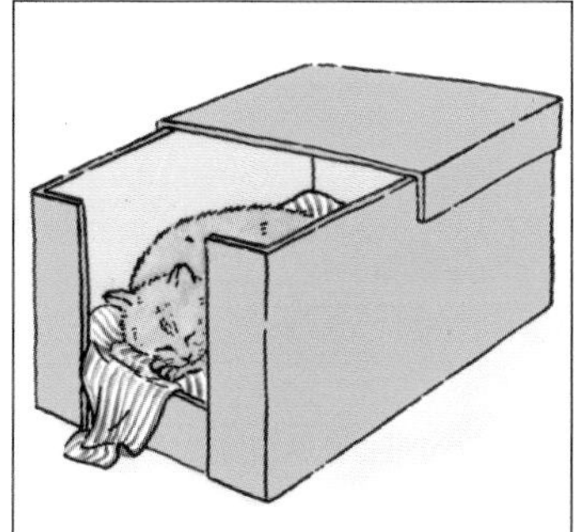

2) The kittening box consists of a cardboard box with a removable lid.

Rearing by a Foster Mother

Now and then it happens that the queen—because of a genetic predisposition, a hormonal disorder, or an illness—produces no milk or insufficient milk. If the litter is overly large or if the queen dies or lacks the proper maternal instinct, human intervention and assistance become necessary.

The easiest method of rearing the kittens is to rely on a surrogate. Candidates for the role include cats that have small litters or cats whose young are old enough to be weaned. Usually a queen will readily foster strange kittens if you first put them in her nest with her young and let her return to them about an hour later under supervision.

Rearing Orphaned Kittens

If you can't find a surrogate, you will have to rear the kittens yourself (see illustration, page 43). Special pet nursers are available (in pet stores) for that purpose.

Housing: Put the cardboard box in a warm, draft-free place and line it with an absorbent terrycloth towel. During the first and second weeks of the kittens' life, use an infrared lamp to provide the necessary warmth: 85°F (30°C). At the beginning of the sixth week, reduce the temperature to 68°F (20°C).

Milk replacer: Cows' milk does not contain enough fat and protein for the little kittens. Use a special queen's milk replacer available in powdered or liquid form (in pet stores). Mix the powdered form with boiled water according to the manufacturer's instructions.

Feeding: Especially during the first few days, the kittens have to be fed every two hours around the clock. Heat the milk replacer to 100.4°F (38°C), place a kitten belly-down on your lap, and gently place one hand around its neck. Then slowly push the nipple of the pet nurser into the kitten's tiny mouth. After every feeding, lightly massage the kitten's little abdomen and excretory organs with a damp cloth in order to stimulate digestion and elimination. Wipe the excretory organs clean with a damp cloth.

Weaning: From the fourth week on start getting the kittens used to solid food. Place ½ teaspoonful of strained baby cereal and some meat juice or consommé along with milk replacer in a bowl. Gradually increase the proportion of solid food until the eighth week, the time when normally reared kittens are weaned by their mothers.

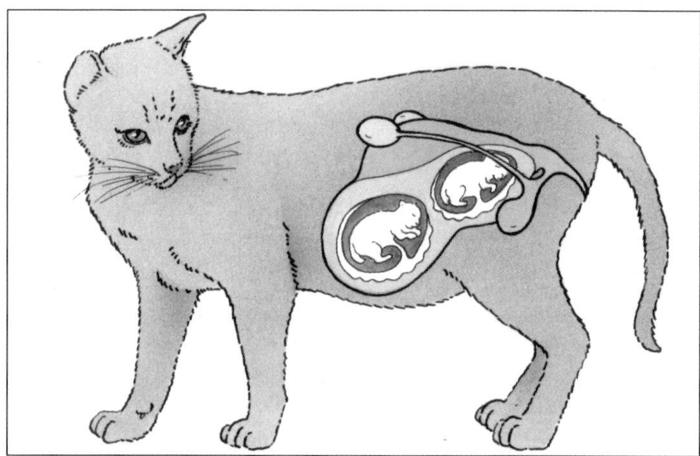

3) The unborn kittens (fetuses) in their mother's body: On the day they are born they are about 5 inches (13 cm) long.

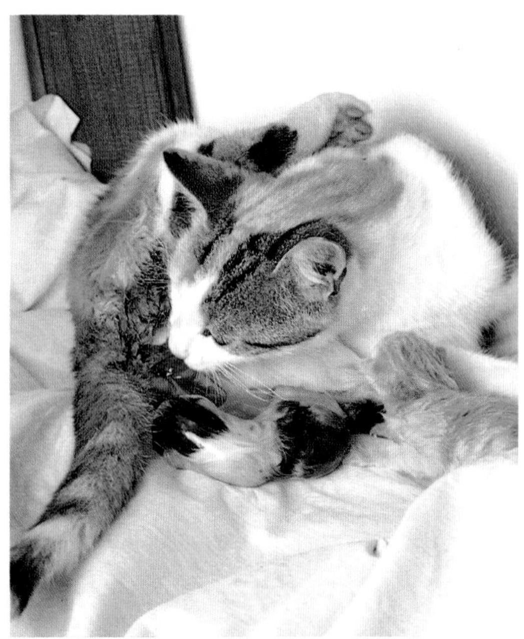

The mother cleans the birth opening . . .

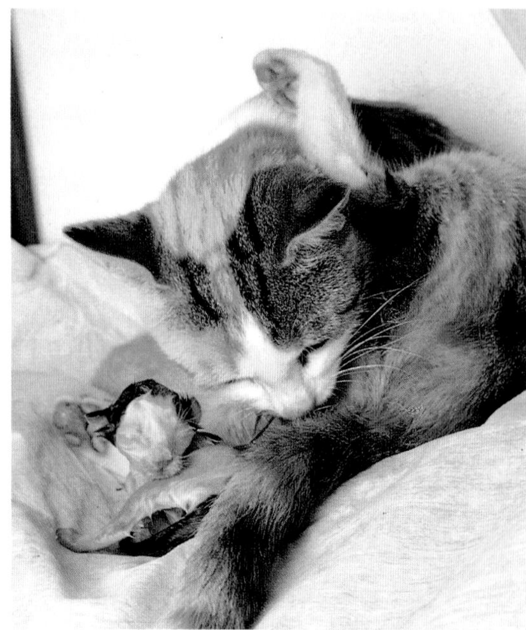

. . . and frees the kitten from the amniotic sac.

in her nipples. Normally a rather pale skin color, they begin to turn pink and become firmer and raised. The cat's abdomen does not become visibly rounder until about 30 days after conception. During the final three weeks of pregnancy, you often can feel or even see the kittens move.

The veterinarian can diagnose pregnancy by palpation around the third week. From the 50th day on, the veterinarian can x-radiograph the queen to provide you with information about the kittens in the womb (see illustration, page 39).

The average duration of pregnancy is 63 to 64 days, but fluctuations of up to six days more or less are completely within the normal range.

The Course of Labor

Independent cats withdraw to a protected spot to give birth, while cats that have a close relationship to a human will accept that person's help and willingly use the kittening box set up for them (see "How-to: Kittening," page 38). Labor can be divided into various stages: the preliminary stage, the dilatation stage, and the expulsive stage, in addition to the afterbirth stage.

The preliminary stage: The only external signs are swelling in the vaginal area, swelling of the nipples, and odd behavior on the female's part. Days before giving birth she becomes restless and goes to the kittening box with increasing frequency. Shortly before delivery she scrapes in the box, lies down in it for a brief time, runs to her litter box but does not use it, and then resumes her restless wandering about.

Sit down next to the kittening box and speak soothingly to your cat. As you stroke her belly, you will clearly feel the movements of the unborn kittens.

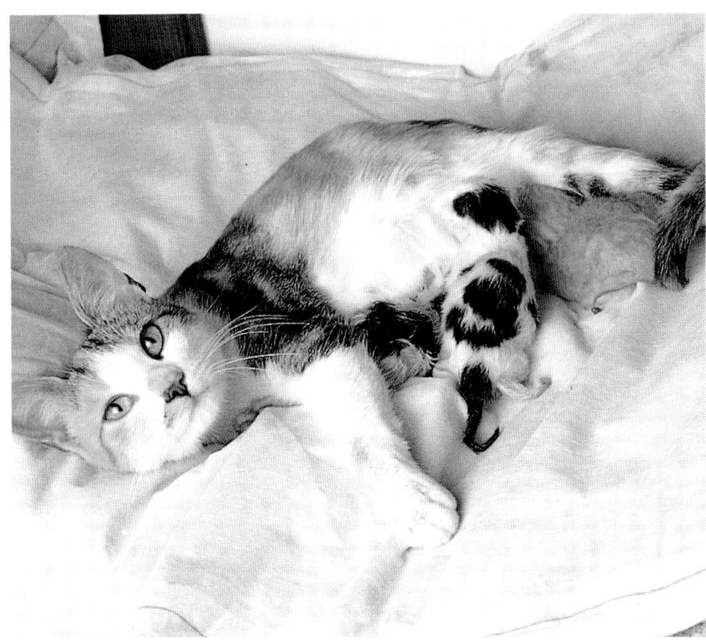

The kittens single-mindedly hunt for their mother's teats.

The period of dilatation: This stage of labor can last one or two hours. The birth canal gradually becomes wider, and clear mucus is discharged. Two or three hours after the first labor pain, you can expect to see the first kitten.

The expulsive stage of delivery: If this is your cat's first litter, the expulsion of the first kitten is usually arduous and can take an hour. In a squatting position or lying on her side, the queen squeezes the kitten out. The subsequent births are less difficult. Cats give birth to as many as eight kittens, in rare instances even more. Normally, parturition is concluded three to six hours after the first kitten has made its appearance. With older females as well as some purebreds the process often can take longer.

The afterbirth stage: The mother should free each newborn kitten from the fetal membranes and lick it dry. In this way she also stimulates the young animal's respiration, intestinal function, and locomotor activity. When the afterbirth is expelled, most mothers bite through the kitten's umbilical cord and consume it along with the afterbirth, which contains vital nutrients and minerals.

If the mother does not free the newborn kitten from the fetal membranes at once, you will have to do it for her or the kitten will suffocate. The membrane should break and peel away easily if you rub the top of the kitten's skull gently with a clean finger or a small piece of clean cloth. If the membrane breaks, peel it away from the kitten's face. If the membrane does not break, pinch it between your thumb and forefinger at the base of the kitten's skull and pull it away from the skull carefully until the membrane tears, then remove it from the kitten's face.

The regenerative stage: The expanded uterus slowly shrinks to its normal size. Usually a reddish-brown vaginal discharge is evident, later becoming lighter in color.

Estrus in the mother cat is suppressed naturally for the time being by milk production for her nursing young. If you want to make sure there are no further offspring, spay your pet as soon as her kittens have gone to their new homes (see "Altering or Sterilization," page 24).

Complications During Labor

Responsible cat owners need to supervise their pets during labor because owners must react immediately if complications arise. Right before the delivery alert your veterinarian, so that he or she can come to your aid if need be.

Difficult labor usually announces itself by unsuccessful pushing and straining. At other times problems are recognizable by overly long intervals (several hours) between the births of the individual kittens (for example, in the case of poor contractions).

- It can happen that a kitten is in an abnormal presentation or gets stuck in the birth canal because of the kitten's large size. Here only veterinary surgery can help. A Caesarean section often is the surest way to help the cat.
- A veterinarian's assistance is also necessary if you observe a discolored, foul-smelling vaginal discharge, or if the mother cat lies apathetically in the kittening box after giving birth and pays no attention to her young.
- Normally the cat severs the kitten's umbilical cord by biting it in two. Among purebred cats, however, this behavior sometimes is diminished. Then human intervention is necessary to help the cat. To keep from injuring the newborn's abdomen, firmly grasp the umbilical cord 4 to 6 inches from the body and carefully cut off the projecting portion with sterilized scissors.

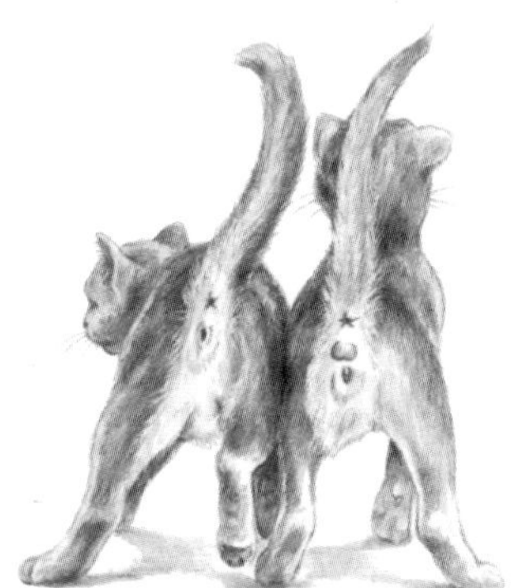

Sex differences between the female (left) and the male (right).

Postpartum Disorders

Delivery can be followed by heavy, prolonged vaginal bleeding. Especially after an unborn kitten or a placenta has been retained in the queen's body, a seriously diseased state results, manifesting itself initially as fever, refusal to eat, extreme thirst, lack of milk, and neglect of her young. In every case it is essential to consult your veterinarian without delay.

Eclampsia

Cats, too, can occasionally suffer from eclampsia—sudden development of convulsions—brought on by a lack of calcium in their blood. This can occur shortly before birth or in the first four weeks after birth. This life-threatening condition has to be remedied immediately by veterinary medical treatment (calcium infusions).

Inadequate Milk Supply

Insufficient production of milk can have a variety of causes:

- hormonal disorders
- postpartum infection
- inflammation of the cat's breasts

In every case treatment by a veterinarian is necessary. With inflammation of the breasts, the only symptom the cat owner notices is that the mother cat cuffs her young to keep them away when they want to nurse. Such inflammations are rare in cats, however.

Often, adequate milk production in the mother cat does not begin on time. Then the young have to be raised by a surrogate or with your help (see "How-to: Kittening," page 38).

Development of Kittens

The normal weight of the newborns ranges from 3.2 to 3.9 ounces (90 to 110 g). Kittens are nidiculous animals: They are born blind and deaf. They already possess a well-developed sense of smell, however. Before their mother has finished licking them dry, they already are searching single-mindedly for the milk-dispensing teat. With large litters in particular, the newborns fight long and hard for a good spot at their mother's breasts and try to push their rivals away with their heads and tiny paws.

You can tell the kittens' sex in the following way: The distance between the anus and the genital opening is greater in a male than in a female. The male's genital opening is round, the female's, oval (see drawing, left).

In the first few days the kittens' specially designed tongues enclose the much-sought-after nipple like a tube.

The little kittens don't let go even when they are asleep. Often they continue to cling to their mother when she leaves the kittening box. Their kneading—pushing their front paws in alternation against her side when they suckle—stimulates her flow of milk. The mother cat uses her tongue to massage her babies' abdomens and anal regions, simultaneously ingesting their excreted matter as she does, to keep the kittening box clean. Not until the second or third day does the mother leave the box for a short time to eat and to use the litter box. During the next few days she frequently tries to move her entire litter to new nursery quarters. To do so, she carries each kitten by the nape of its neck, firmly held in her mouth but unharmed by her teeth. The kitten allows itself to go totally limp.

Between the eighth and the twelfth days the eyelids open, and the young kittens blink at the light of day for the first time. At roughly the same time, their first milk teeth erupt from their gums.

In the fourth week the kittens, still clumsy, start to play.

From the fourth week on the little kittens can become accustomed to mushy and semisolid food, which makes them increasingly less reliant on their mother's milk. Baby cats also thoroughly enjoy gruel made with milk. To make oatmeal gruel, mix three tablespoons instant oatmeal for infants, one teaspoon yeast flakes, one egg yolk, and one cup warm milk (but no sugar). Commercial kitten food is also available. Keep an eye on the kittens' digestion: Milk can induce diarrhea (see page 85).

In the fourth and fifth weeks the righting reflex develops—the ability to land on all fours after a fall. Strangers are greeted by hissing and laid-back ears. Playing turns into boisterous romping and imaginative acrobatics. As soon as the kittens leave the kittening box on their own, you need to provide a shallow litter box for them (see "How-to: Kittening," page 38).

Between the sixth and the ninth weeks the kittens already are capable of doing a great deal, including arching their backs, chasing each other, jumping, washing themselves, and using the litter box. All their milk teeth are in, and they are eating on their own. Many mother cats now begin to ward off attempts to nurse by giving the kitten a blow with their paws.

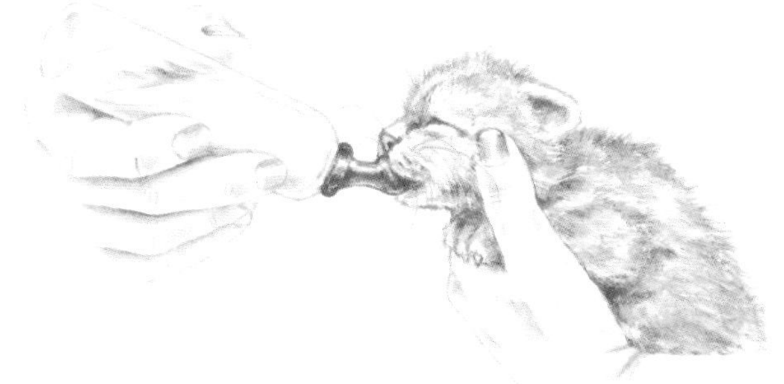

There are special pet nursers for hand-rearing.

Finding Homes for the Kittens

At the age of 12 weeks the kittens are ready to move to their new homes. By this time they have been dewormed and have received the first of the requisite shots (see "Vaccination Schedule for Preventive Health Care," page 26).

Kittens that are separated from their mothers earlier than this often fail to thrive for the rest of their lives. Give your kittens only to people whom you know well and who are reliable and fond of animals. To find buyers for purebred kittens, you can advertise the little animals for sale in specialized magazines for cat fanciers, for example. Often the local breed societies can help by acting as an intermediary (see "Information," page 126).

The Old Cat

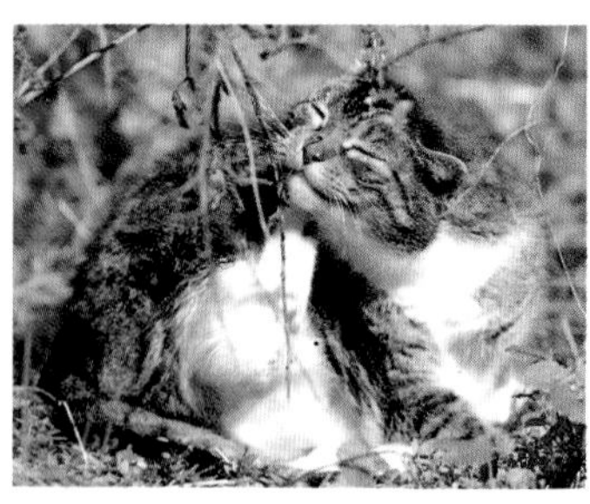

It is by no means inevitable that your cat's health will suffer with increasing age. Often the symptoms that herald the end of a cat's life (weight loss, apathy, diarrhea or constipation, and neglect of coat grooming) first appear only in very advanced age. When your cat gets old, it needs your attention in special measure. Its environment should change as little as possible at this time. A new kitten in the family probably would be annoying to your old pet.

Taking Care of an Old Cat

Where grooming is concerned, old cats need the assistance of their humans. Because old cats no longer wash themselves so thoroughly, dirty areas of the coat have to be cleaned with a damp cloth (see "How-to: Preventive Care," page 14). Your care should include periodically feeling your pet's body to see whether lumps and tumors are present. Only early detection makes it possible for the veterinarian's help to be effective. Many old indoor cats use their scratching posts less often. You need to check their nails more frequently and, if necessary, trim them or have them trimmed by the veterinarian (see photos, page 24). Regular vaccinations, deworming, and check-ups by the veterinarian should remain a part of your pet's health care, especially when it is old (see page 23).

Tips on Feeding

It is entirely normal for very old cats to lose weight. They eat less, and they also are less able to utilize their food than are young animals. Go ahead and encourage your cat to eat by offering it treats. There is cause for alarm, however, if you cat loses weight rapidly and displays other symptoms as well (see "Cats That Are Skin and Bones," page 21). Then it is time to consult a veterinarian.

The following are a few tips on feeding your old cat:

- An old cat (more than 15 years old) should be fed its daily ration in three or four servings spread over the course of the day.
- Feed your pet protein of high nutritive value, present in plentiful amounts in commercial cat food, fish, meat, organ meats, and poultry. (Canned cat food is best for old cats.)
- From time to time mix 1 teaspoonful of butter or margarine into the food to give the cat additional calories.
- Now and then add some commercial cat laxative to the food to prevent constipation. Bran and fish with a high fat content also aid digestion.

Hint: Because old cats very often have bad teeth or no teeth at all, you need to cut their food into small pieces before serving.

Diseases of Old Age

In old age the efficiency and regenerative power of the organs diminish. Diseases increase as a result. Many of the cat's sensory capacities, including hearing and sight, can become poorer in old age.

Dental problems: Dental problems rank first among the problems of old age. Holes develop in the teeth; often thick deposits of tartar form on the teeth, and the gums may become inflamed (see page 68). Frequently the veterinarian has to extract diseased teeth.

Intestinal problems: Old cats often suffer from sluggishness of the bowels and constipation (see page 86). A commercially available cat laxative may solve the problem. If constipation is severe, the veterinarian can give your pet an enema (see photo, page 89). Some old cats also suffer from chronic diarrhea. Usually this is an indication of a serious illness.

Joint problems: Old cats can become lame as a result of wear and tear on a joint (see page 72). In such cases the veterinarian will give your pet anti-inflammatory medications.

Tumors: Tumorous disorders become increasingly frequent with advancing age, and they are often the cause of death in old cats. In principle, tumor cells, which arise from normal body cells, can appear in any tissue or organ of the body. Their appearance may be triggered by infections, genetic factors, or environmental factors.

Tumor cells damage the organism not only by utilizing vital substances but also by releasing their own metabolic products. Principally, however, they damage vital cells and organs and can also cause serious disturbances of hormonal balance or immune resistance. If a tumor's growth is limited and localized and no secondary tumors (metastases) develop, we describe it as benign. Unchecked growth and the tendency to invade the organism with metastases are characteristics of a malignant tumor. Tumors generally can be classified accurately only by examination of tissue by histopathology.

Euthanasia

If a cat is unable to live free of pain after a traffic accident or as a result of an incurable disease or an age-related infirmity, you should have the veterinarian put your pet to sleep with an intravenous injection of an anesthetic agent. The cat will feel nothing and will go to sleep peacefully.

The veterinarian will advise euthanizing an animal only after weighing all the circumstances. After so many years of close attachment, you may want to accompany your cat to the veterinarian's office and stay with your pet when it receives the injection that delivers it from its suffering.

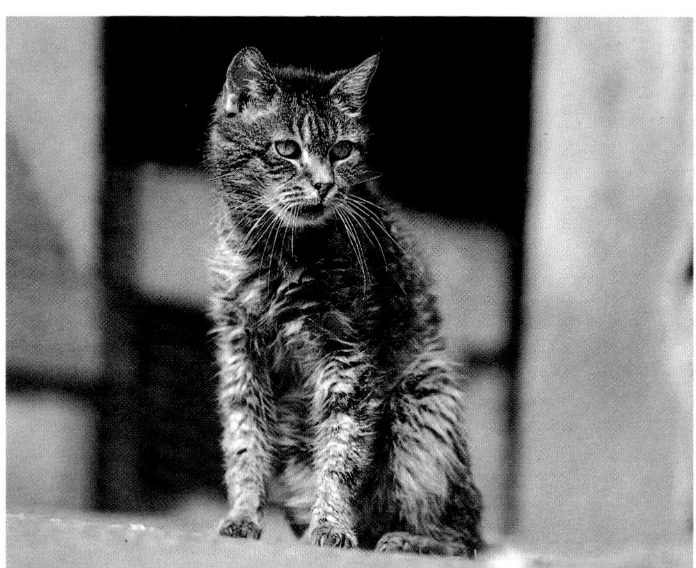

The coat of an old cat is no longer smooth and glossy.

Dangers for Cats and Owners

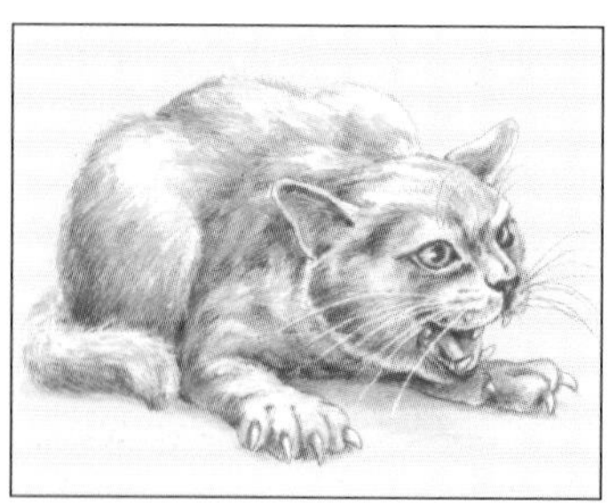

There are a number of pathogens that can attack both cats and humans. If an indoor cat is dewormed and vaccinated, and if it is given only cooked food or commercial cat food, then it rarely will become infected with pathogens that are potentially dangerous to you. Outdoor cats will present less risk for human health, provided a few precautionary measures are taken.

Infections and Parasites

Some carriers of infection and parasites can attack several animal species. If a human becomes infected, we call the disease a zoonosis (see "Glossary," page 113). In the material below we list the most important diseases and parasites that are communicable to humans (see "Information," page 126).

Rabies: A viral disease that is communicable to other animals and to humans by the bite of a rabid animal (see page 108). Every cat that is allowed to roam outdoors, is shown at pedigreed cat shows, or goes with you on trips abroad has to be vaccinated against rabies (see "Vaccination Schedule for Preventive Health Care," page 26). A human can be given immunity by injections, even immediately after infection occurs.

Pox virus infection in cats: A very rare viral disease that is transmitted to cats by their prey and to humans by cats (see page 105). Especially at risk are children, the elderly, and people with weakened immune systems.

Bacterial infections: In rare instances diseases (see page 110) caused by bacteria (for example, chlamydia and salmonella) can be communicated to humans by cats. In people with lowered resistance, salmonella can occasionally cause serious disease. If a cat has salmonella, strict precautionary measures are necessary (for example, wearing gloves when you clean the cat's litter box).

Fungal infections: Skin fungi are easily communicable to humans (see pages 76 and 111). If your cat is affected, practice good hygiene, and wash your hands after touching your pet. Fungal infections that affect the respiratory organs, mucous membranes, and intestinal tract (systemic mycosis) are rare. Nonetheless, it is conceivable that these fungi, which cause serious diseases, could be transmitted to humans (see page 111). Treatment with antifungal drugs is protracted.

Toxoplasmosis: Caused by parasites that use many animal species as well as man as intermediate hosts (see page 97). After infection, the cat passes the pathogen in its stool for a period of seven to 14 days. Remove the feces at once (wear rubber gloves) in order to avert the danger of transmission to humans.

Toxoplasmosis can be dangerous for pregnant women. When primary infection occurs, the pathogens sometimes induce miscarriages or damage the unborn child. Women should have themselves tested in early pregnancy to determine whether they have ever had toxoplasmosis. After recovery from the infection both humans and animals are immune to the pathogen.

Intestinal worms: Hookworm larvae (see page 101) penetrate the skin and cause skin reactions in humans. At risk are children who play bare-armed and bare-legged in damp areas.

Roundworm eggs (see page 100) are excreted in cats' feces. Children can become infected when they come in contact with buried cat droppings while playing in a sandbox.

Tapeworms: The fox tapeworm (see page 102) is of importance. Humans also can be infected by the dangerous bladder worm (*Cysticercus*) through contact with worm eggs from cat feces.

Fleas, mites, and ticks: Cat fleas (see page 98) attack humans only temporarily but cause severe itching. If your cat is infested with fleas, treat it with a gel or a powder, disinfect the surroundings with parasite spray, and vacuum your home thoroughly. Flea eggs can survive for as long as 12 months, especially in carpet pile and floorboard crevices.

Burrowing mites (see page 97) in rare instances are transmitted to humans and cause symptoms of mange (scabies). If your cat is affected, treat it with appropriate remedies and give the places it frequents a thorough cleaning.

Ticks (see page 99) potentially can transmit borreliosis (see "Glossary," page 113) or Lyme disease to humans (cats are not affected) or cause meningitis. If you find a tick on your cat, remove it at once with tick tweezers (see photo, page 100).

Scratches

When you deal with cats, bites and scratches can occur. There is the danger of a wound becoming infected, which can turn into a serious, festering inflammation, blood poisoning (sepsis), or tetanus. It is also possible to contract rabies through a bite (see page 108).

Use a topical disinfectant on superficial injuries. If there is any doubt, it is essential to consult a physician. Preventive vaccinations against tetanus are advisable for humans.

Allergies

Many people are allergic to a host of substances in their environments. Some people are allergic to cat hair. If tests prove that you have an irremediable allergy to cats, avoid contact with cats in the future.

Pets Are Soul Food

The health risk that cats present is worth noting, of course, but overall it is to be regarded as relatively minor. On the other hand, you need to keep in mind the substantial health benefits that humans derive from the animals with which they share their lives. Domesticated animals, particularly house pets like dogs and cats, fulfill, in an uncomplicated way, our need for physical contact and solicitude. Medical research confirms that physical and mental problems—including the risk of a heart attack and depression—can be decidedly improved by keeping a pet cat, for example. Pets are especially important for lonely children and elderly people.

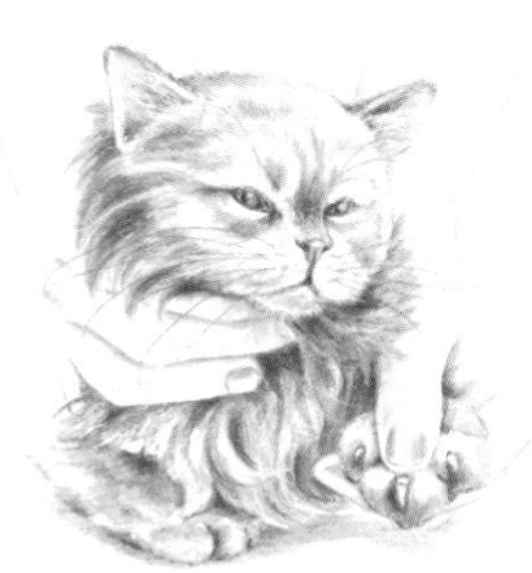

When handling a cat, you can get scratched.

Visiting the Veterinarian

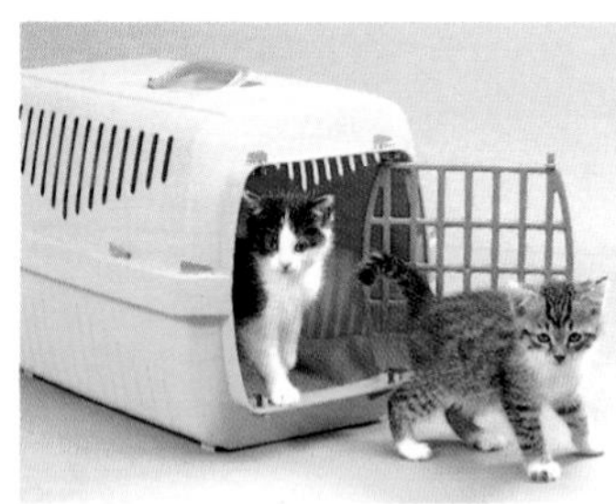

Don't wait until your cat shows obvious symptoms of disease to take it to the veterinarian. You also need the veterinarian's help with your pet's preventive health care program when vaccinations are due or deworming is necessary. Consequently, you need to find a veterinarian who can deal well with cats and whom you can trust. The choice of a veterinarian will be easier for you if you consult other cat owners.

The Veterinarian's Office

Generally, cats are brought to the veterinarian's office for examination and treatment. House calls by a veterinarian are the exception rather than the rule. The cat should be transported in a container that can be securely closed (carrier, basket, cage). If need be, you also can use a sturdy cardboard box. Get the cat used to the carrier before the first trip to the veterinarian so that the cat feels comfortable in the carrier and does not get agitated unnecessarily. Leave your pet in its container while you wait in the office; remove the cat only for purposes of examination and treatment. That will prevent conflicts with other animals in the veterinarian's waiting room.

Important: If your cat has serious injuries (see "How-to: First Aid for Cats," page 54), you need to be especially careful when transporting it.

The Examination

Information about the cat's age, care, previous illnesses, and behavior is important for the veterinarian. Describe the symptoms as accurately as possible. Making notes of what you have observed is helpful. Use the following checklist:

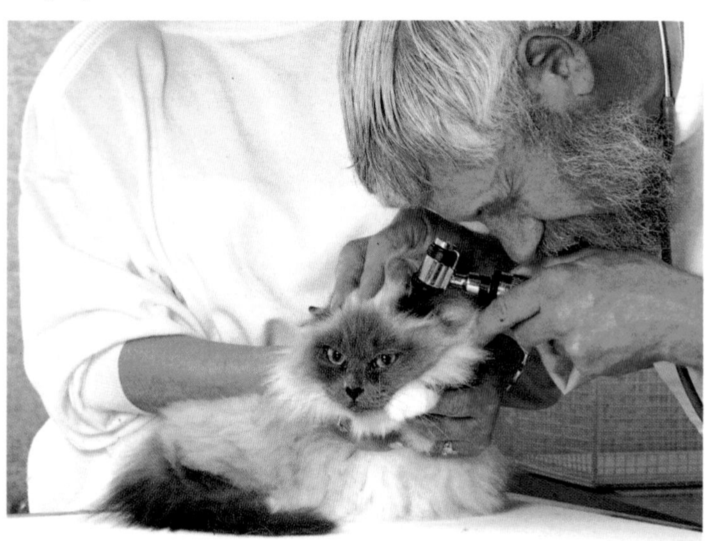

Ear check: Mites can cause inflammations.

- Does the cat have a healthy appetite, or does it refuse to eat?
- Does it have diarrhea or constipation?
- Does it vomit more than usual? How often?
- Does it drink more water than usual?
- Does it have a fever (see page 50)?
- Does it repeatedly shake its head and scratch at its ears?
- Does it behave differently; for example, is it apathetic?
- Does it fail to use the litter box, and does it neglect its grooming?
- Does it have any pain when touched?

Important: Bring along stool and vomitus samples. Don't forget the vaccination record.

If anesthesia is scheduled don't let the cat have anything to eat on the day of the procedure (see "Anesthesia," page 52).

During the examination the pet owner's help is not needed because a staff assistant will hold the cat understandingly. With operations, too, the owner's presence is not advisable. When the treatment is over, the veterinarian will discuss with you the further course of action, possibly schedule another visit, and give you medications and directions for treatment.

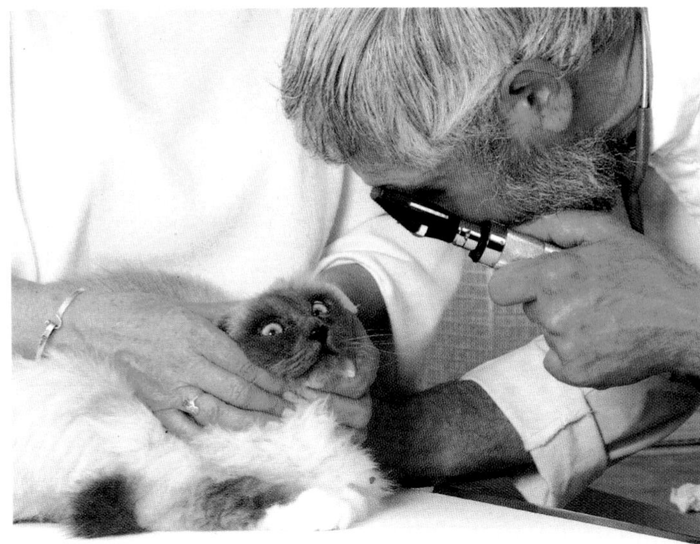

The veterinarian looks at the eyes with a special instrument.

The Cat as Patient

As a rule the carrier with the cat inside is placed on the examining table, and the cat is taken out only when everything is in readiness for the examination. As patients most cats are agreeable and calm. They readily allow themselves to be handled if they are dealt with gently, held without exertion of much pressure, stroked, and grasped by the shoulders. Even injections, the drawing of blood samples, examination of the oral cavity, and ear treatments can be performed without resistance.

If the cat resists: Now and then it happens that cats allow themselves to be handled only with great difficulty, or not at all. Some resist from the outset out of fear. Others become increasingly fearful and mistrustful only after unpleasant experiences in the veterinarian's office.

If your pet has repeatedly proved very hard to handle in the veterinarian's office, before a scheduled visit you can add a tranquilizer (obtainable from the veterinarian) to the cat's food. Sometimes a tranquilizer or an anesthetic has to be injected before the veterinarian is able to attempt any examination and treatment at all.

Nursing a Sick Cat

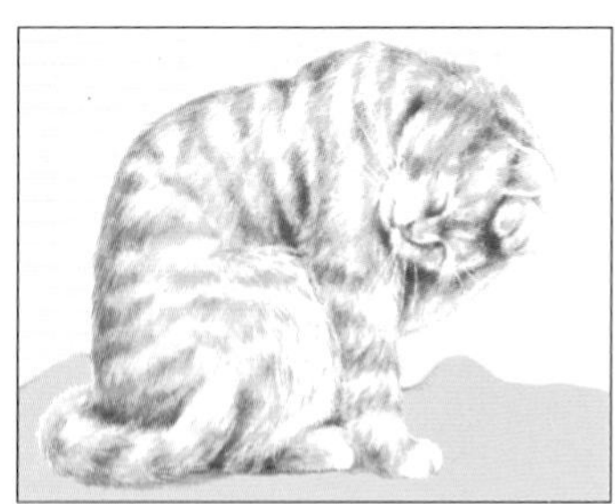

When a sick cat is on the mend, two factors are extremely important: comfortable quarters and sympathetic attention from familiar humans. For this reason you need to speak soothingly to your pet and stroke it from time to time. If continued treatment at home is required, you need to carry out the veterinarian's instructions to the letter.

The Sickbed

With many diseases it is advisable to leave the cat indoors for a few days. Sick cats have to be protected from damp, cold weather in particular. Fix a warm sickbed for your pet by putting a hot water bottle in the basket where the cat sleeps or in a cardboard box. Lay a blanket over the hot water bottle, and place the cat on that (see illustration, page 51). Make sure the basket or box is free from drafts, and put it in a quiet, familiar spot.

Hint: If other cats live in your household, a sick pet with a contagious disease has to be isolated (see "Dangers for Cats and Owners," page 46, and "Information," page 126).

Feeding a Sick Cat

If your cat lacks appetite, offer it fresh, slightly warmed tidbits or tasty food concentrates (available from veterinarians). If your cat cannot chew well, puree the pieces of food. Sometimes, daubing food on your pet's nose will stimulate his appetite. If the cat cannot eat on its own for a prolonged period, it has to be fed. Using a disposable syringe without a needle, trickle meat or chicken broth (unseasoned) into the cat's mouth from one side.

Force feeding is not necessary as a rule; it does little good and sometimes even causes the cat pain, which leads to mistrust of humans.

Fresh drinking water has to be within reach at all times because a continuous intake of fluids is very important for a sick cat. Make sure your pet is drinking enough. If it is not doing so on its own, you have to instill water into the cat by means of a syringe (without a needle).

Hint: Many illnesses, especially diarrhea and vomiting, result in dehydration of the organism, which is treated by the veterinarian with infusions of electrolyte solutions (see "Glossary," page 113).

Taking the Cat's Temperature

The following method for taking the cat's temperature works best with two people. One person should hold the cat's shoulders and front paws firmly while the other should take its temperature. To do so, raise the cat's tail slightly and insert the thermometer, lubricated with a little petroleum jelly, into its anus horizontally (see photo, page 93). A conventional thermometer has to remain in the rectum for about two minutes, while a digital thermometer will give an accurate readout after one minute. While you are taking the cat's temperature, talk to the cat and stroke it.

The normal temperature ranges between 100 and 103°F (37.8–39.2°C). Subnormal temperature, as well as elevated temperature, can be a sign of illness.

Coat Care

If the cat is so ill that it no longer is able to wash itself, you have to clean its coat with a damp cloth after meals and after passage of stool. If your pet is not in pain, it is all right to brush its coat carefully as well (see "How-to: Preventive Care," page 14).

Giving Your Pet Medications

Administering medications is often not easy. Just how difficult it turns out to be depends on the nature of the medicine, the personality of the cat, and the dexterity of the owner.

Tablets, pills, and capsules: If the cat still has a good appetite, the tablet can be concealed in a tasty bit of food (larger tablets can be broken up and divided among several pieces of food). If the cat knows what you are up to, however, the following method will help: Using the thumb and forefinger of one hand, hold the tablet ready to use. Place your other hand on the cat's head, right behind its teeth, and exert a slight pressure. That will cause your pet to open its jaws involuntarily. Next, place the tablet as far back on the tongue as possible. Finally, hold the cat's little mouth closed. With one hand, gently massage its throat in an upward direction, so that the cat will swallow the tablet (see photos, page 60).

Liquid medications: It is best to administer them with a disposable syringe (available from the veterinarian) without the needle (see illustration, page 27). To do so, raise the cat's head slightly and empty the contents of the syringe into the cat's mouth at one side, behind the eyeteeth—but not in one gush; otherwise, the cat will choke. You also can trickle drops directly onto a paw. The cat will lick them off automatically—provided they don't taste too bitter.

Eye Ointments and Drops

With eye diseases, it frequently is necessary to treat the cat with ointment or drops.

Applying eye ointment: Hold the back of the cat's head firmly with one hand, carefully drawing back the upper eyelid with your index finger. Then, with your other hand, place a ribbon of ointment about one-fifth of an inch (5 mm) long beneath the lid. Never touch the eyeball directly with the tip of the tube.

Putting in eye drops: To put drops in your pet's eye, hold the back of its head firmly, raise its head, and carefully pull back the lower eyelid with your index finger. With the eyedropper, introduce two or three drops behind the lid. Never touch the eyeball directly!

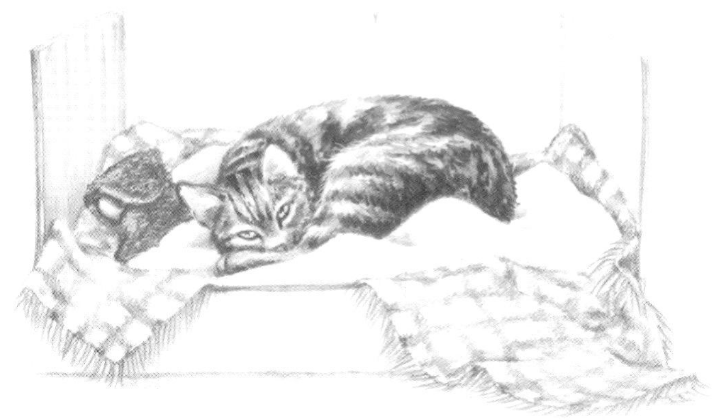

A sick cat needs plenty of sleep and proper care.

Ear Drops

Gently pull up the cat's ear flap (external ear) until the auditory canal is open. Then put four or five drops into the ear. Next, gently massage the base of the ear in front to distribute the liquid inside the ear canal.

Inhalations

With diseases of the respiratory passages (see page 90), you can give your cat an inhalation to relieve its discomfort. Prepare a hot chamomile infusion with chamomile concentrate. Place the cat in a carrier that can be latched (see photo, page 48). Put a bowl containing the infusion in front of the carrier opening, and, using a towel, fan the hot vapors into the interior, so that the cat will inhale them.

Insulin Injections

If your cat is diabetic (see page 79), you need to lower its blood sugar level by giving it a daily insulin injection. The veterinarian will provide you with a syringe and needle and also show you how to administer the injection.

It is best to give the injection in the nape of the neck or the back area. With one hand pull up the cat's skin to form a "tent." With the other take the syringe and stick the needle into the hollow area beneath the top of the tent. Then let go of the skin. The tip of the needle has to remain under the skin. Push the plunger into the syringe, thereby injecting the insulin subcutaneously.

Hint: Insert the needle at a different spot each time you give an injection.

Anesthesia

Before anesthesia: If anesthesia is to be administered—during surgery or even during tartar removal—don't let your pet eat anything in the 12 hours preceding the scheduled procedure.

After anesthesia: If the cat has had surgery, you generally are not allowed to take it back home until it has come out of the anesthesia. If it continues to sleep, which occurs with old or fat cats, it has to be protected against hypothermia during the trip home and after arrival there. Wrap your pet in a blanket and, after returning home, lay a hot water bottle beneath it. Check your cat's respiration and pulse (see "Health Check," page 11).

Baths for Skin Infections

If your cat is infested with dermatophytes—fungi parasitic on the skin—it can be treated with a fungicide (see "Glossary," page 113), which usually has to be dissolved in water. Before bathing your cat, put cotton in its ears to keep the water out. Next, wet only its coat, and massage it lightly. Place one hand over your pet's eyes for protection. Rinse with clear water, but don't wash all the medication out of the coat so that it can have an aftereffect. Finally, dry your pet carefully with a towel. Also clean the places where the cat likes to lie, and wash blankets and pillows.

Hint: Remember that antifungal pet shampoos have active ingredients. Wash your hands thoroughly after bathing the cat. If your skin is sensitive or if you have allergic tendencies, wear disposable gloves (see "Important Notes," page 127).

A Home Medical Kit

To be prepared for emergencies you should put together a small home medical kit for your pet. The instruments it should include are:

- thermometer
- tweezers
- tick tweezers
- nail clippers
- three plastic syringes (without needles)—with fill volumes of 2, 5, and 10 milliliters, respectively—to give your pet medications, nourishment, and liquids
- curved scissors with one blunt edge and one sharp edge

The bandaging materials it should include are:

- two elastic gauze bandages, 1.5 inches (4 cm) wide, to dress the paws
- two elastic gauze bandages, 3 inches (8 cm) wide, to dress the head, chest, or abdomen
- one roll of surgical tape
- one package of surgical cotton

The medications it should include will depend on your pet's medical condition. For example, if your cat is diabetic

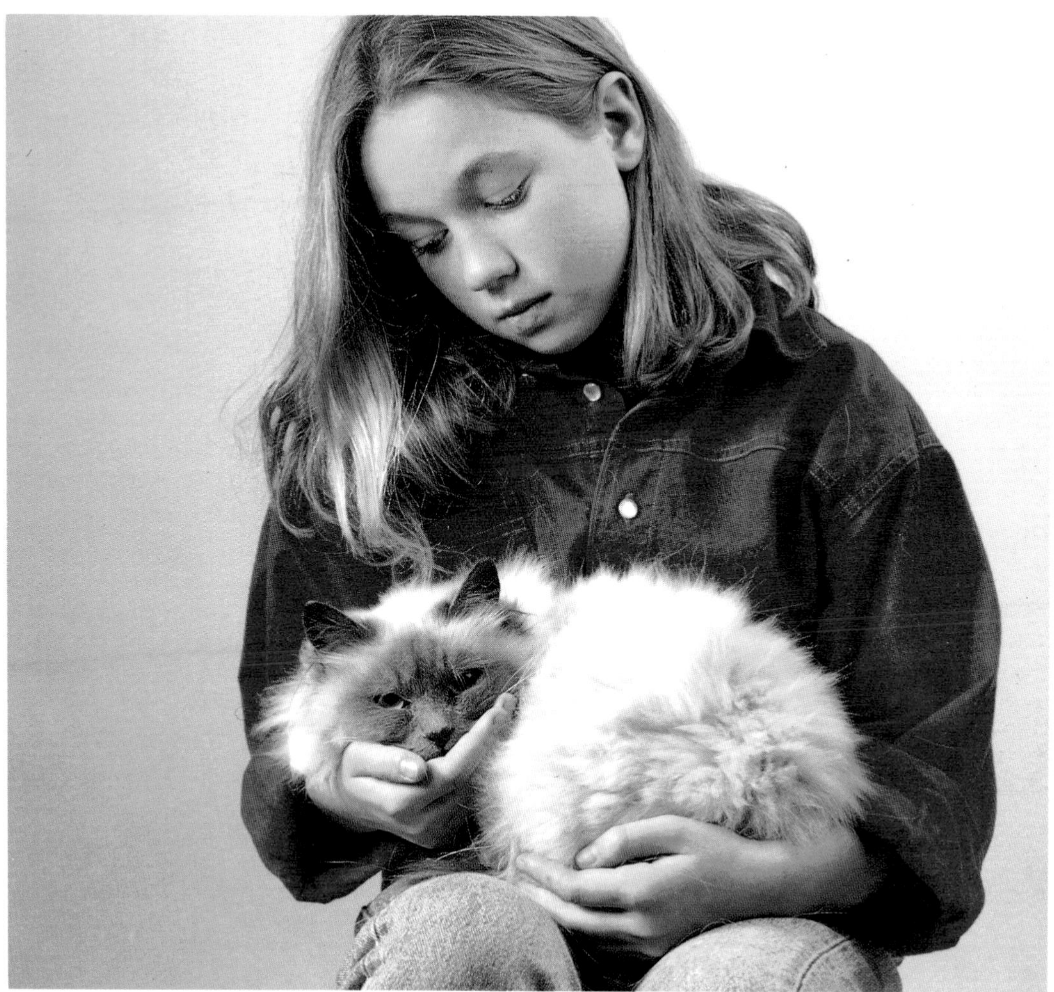

When their pet is ill, children suffer too. This cat is being gently stroked.

(see page 79), keep insulin on hand for its daily injection (store the insulin in the refrigerator).

Hint: Check the expiration date of all medications. If the date has passed, the medication is no longer usable.

Other items the medical kit should include are:

- a bottle of ear-cleaning solution (available from a veterinarian)
- a baby enema to treat constipation
- powder, gel, or spray to control fleas, mites, and ticks (see page 96)

Hint: Exercise extreme caution when using these preparations (see "Information," page 126).

HOW-TO: First Aid for Cats

Potential Dangers to Cats

Cats can be injured by:

- cars or farm machinery (combines, tractors).
- fighting with dogs or other cats.
- being struck on the head, for example, when someone tries to chase the cat away, or by traps that have been set.
- getting entangled (in cords or wire) or getting squeezed (in a tilting window).
- a fall.
- bullets shot by hunters or people who own firearms.

First Aid for Injuries

If the cat is still able to make its way home after being seriously injured, you need to be alert for certain conditions.

Hypothermia can result if the weather is cold or wet. Carefully towel dry the cat.

Behavioral changes such as agitation or disorientation are symptoms of shock. Put the cat in its basket or box and take it to the nearest veterinarian immediately.

Fractures are indicated if the cat limps, if its limbs are in an unnatural position, or if the limbs are abnormally flexible. Here, too, only a veterinarian can help.

Profuse bleeding—after an automobile accident, for example—has to be controlled by a pressure dressing to keep the cat from bleeding to death. To do so, first remove any substantial foreign bodies (rocks, glass, splinters) from the wound. Fold a piece of gauze bandage or clean fabric several times and press it on the wound. Wrap a gauze bandage or an elastic bandage around the affected limb or area. Test the tightness of the dressing by slipping a finger underneath it. If you can do so easily, the dressing is not too tight. Then take the cat to the nearest veterinarian at once.

Poisoning

Poisons can do serious damage to a cat and can bring about its death. Highly toxic substances are harmful even in minute quantities, while other substances produce damage only if ingested frequently or in very large amounts.

Poisons are introduced into the cat's body by way of its tongue (often when it licks its

1) The cat skeleton

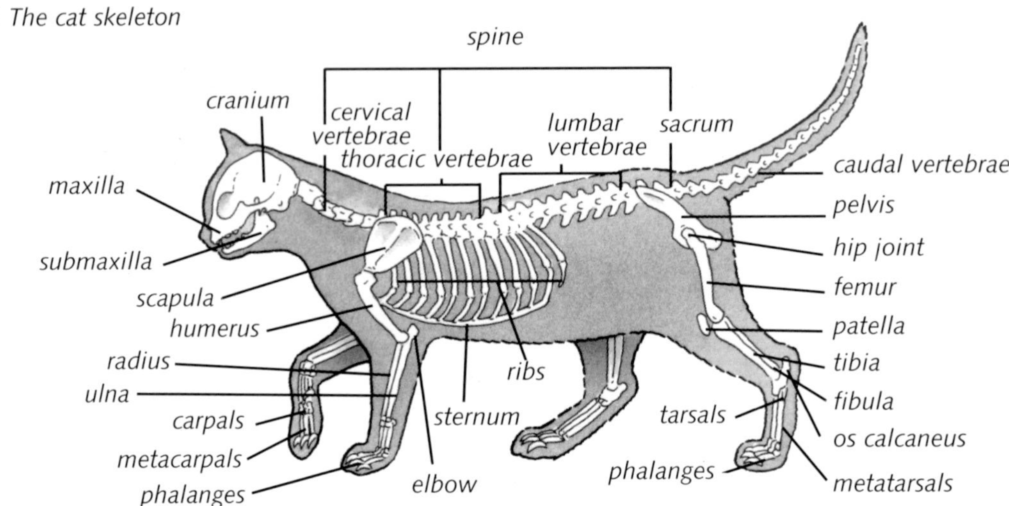

coat), its food, its skin, or the air it breathes.

Symptoms of poisoning may include the following: drooling, vomiting, diarrhea, convulsions, apathy, and loss of consciousness.

In every instance the cat has to be taken to the veterinarian immediately. Generally, it is possible to determine what poison the cat has ingested only if a concrete suspicion exists. If you know what the cat has ingested (e.g., a household product), be sure to bring the container label for the veterinarian to examine. Sometimes a test for that purpose, conducted by a special lab, can provide direct proof.

A veterinarian who knows for sure what the poison is can sometimes administer antidotes. In some cases the cat is also given an emetic.

The Most Common Poisons

Rodent poisons: Poisons that prevent the blood from coagulating (coumarin derivatives) frequently are used as bait to control rats or mice. When rats or mice ingest the poison, profuse internal bleeding results, and the rodents die of internal hemorrhage. If cats eat a fairly large quantity of this poison, they, too, can die of it (see "Nosebleed," page 90).

In addition to the general symptoms of poisoning (see above), coumarin poisoning in a cat can be recognized by bleeding that does not stop,

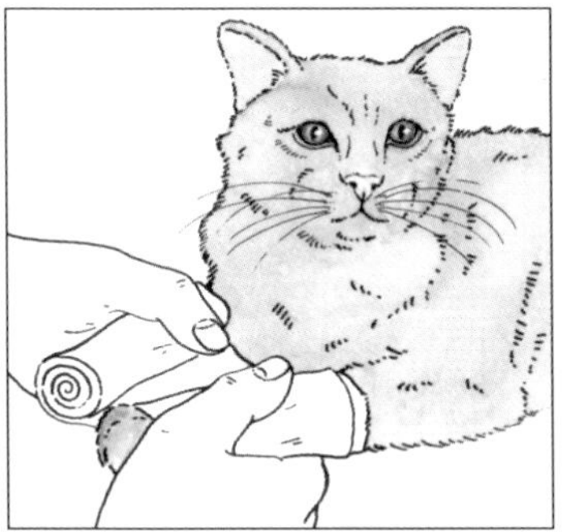

Apply a pressure dressing to profusely bleeding wounds.

hematomas, and pale mucous membranes. If the pet owner notices in time that the cat has been poisoned, the veterinarian can help by giving Vitamin K injections.

Insecticides: Cats have a hypersensitive reaction to chlorinated hydrocarbons and phosphoric acid esters in particular. These toxic substances can be taken in not only by mouth but also through the skin. If there is cause for suspicion, the cat's coat has to be freed immediately of any poison adhering to it (for example, by using dampened paper tissues or by bathing the animal in lukewarm water). Then dry its coat with a towel. Finally, go at once to the veterinarian, who will treat the cat with special antidotes such as atropine and give it infusions to induce the kidneys to eliminate the poison.

Antifreeze (ethylene glycol, glycol): Cats often lick up antifreeze spontaneously because of its sweetish taste. Depending on the amount of poison ingested, serious kidney damage or even kidney failure resulting in death can be the outcome. If you have grounds for suspicion, take your cat to the veterinarian without delay. Ethyl alcohol and sodium hydrocarbonate are used as antidotes. The animal is given an injection to stimulate kidney function.

Petroleum products: Accidents usually happen because fuel oil tanks are not secured properly or because the cat comes into contact with oil spots left by cars. The poison gets into its body not only through the skin but also through the mouth when the cat licks its fur. Clean oil-smeared portions of your pet's coat at once with heated paper tissues or a grease-dissolving agent (a detergent, for example) and water. Take the cat to the veterinarian.

Phytotoxins: Many houseplants contain poisonous substances (see page 10). Before you buy a plant, always find out whether it presents any danger to your cat (see "Information," page 126).

Treating Cat Diseases

What Is Disease?

If a cat owner notices changes in his or her pet, that may be an initial indication of disease.

General symptoms are numerous. Diminished appetite, weight loss, increased girth, sudden behavioral changes, apathy, neglect of grooming, dull coat, hair loss, severe itching, increased elimination of feces and urine, diarrhea, continuous vomiting, increased thirst, or sudden failure to use the litter box.

The causes of disease are manifold. Extreme temperature conditions such as heat, cold, and humidity can promote disease, as can environmental factors that create stress for the cat and weaken its body's defense system—in particular, the keeping of too many cats in too small a space, loneliness, an unhealthy diet, poor care, and insufficient attention. If the environment contains a great many pathogens and if the organism is already weakened, diseases can easily break out.

Healing has to be accomplished by the body with the help of its powers of resistance and renewal. Every living creature is able, in principle, to react to metabolic imbalances in its body, injuries, and infections, and to heal itself in many instances.

If the body's regulatory capacities have been exhausted or if the destructive influence from outside is too great, a turn toward healing often can be achieved only through purposeful treatment by a veterinarian.

In many cases our present understanding in the fields of biology and medicine has made it possible to appraise the cause and course of a disease quite accurately and to administer therapy targeted at it. Great technical advances in diagnostic and therapeutic procedures make it possible to achieve results that were unimaginable only a short while ago. Nevertheless, the

The Anatomy of a Cat

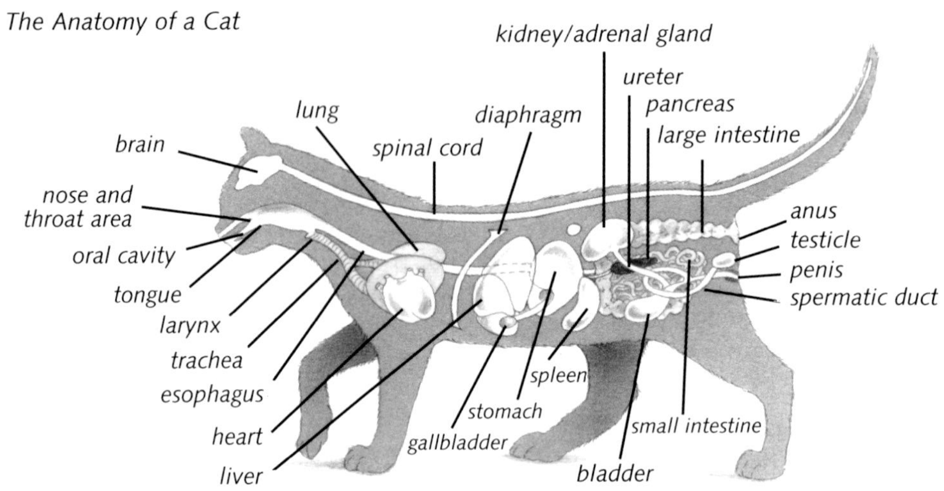

limits of the abilities of science become obvious again and again, even in the field of human medicine.

Naturopathic procedures and homeopathy (see page 58) are applicable to cats as well. Homeopathy can be useful as an adjunct to other therapeutic treatments. The use of homeopathic remedies promotes the animal's powers of self-healing by mobilizing its body's own reserves.

Although the effect of homeopathy cannot be scientifically explained, we repeatedly hear of astonishing recoveries. The body's powers of self-healing also can be stimulated in cats by positive environmental influences and by protection from negative factors. For example, a cat that is extremely ill with symptoms of respiratory disease and dehydration will have a better chance of healing (provided the process is still reversible) if you put it into optimum surroundings without stress rather than in a room crowded with other cats.

How to Use This Book

The diseases described in the following pages are divided into eight sections (on right).

The descriptions of the diseases follow this pattern:

Symptoms: First signs of the disease.

Causes: Triggers of the disease.

Effects: The course the disease may take.

● **Treatment:** What you can do yourself; what the veterinarian will prescribe. An arrow (▶) indicates when professional help is essential.

Follow-up care: What you should do after treatment is terminated.

Prevention: How the disease can be avoided.

Susceptible breeds: Mention of breeds especially vulnerable to the disease.

■ **Homeopathy:** Suggestion of homeopathic remedies you can apply.

Follow-up care, prevention, and susceptible breeds are not always applicable and therefore don't appear in every case.

Homeopathic treatments also are mentioned only if, in the author's opinion, they offer a good chance of success, particularly if used in conjunction with proper veterinary care. Veterinarian Heidrun Gratz, a contributor to this book, has had good experience with these remedies in her practice.

The small picture on the right appears on every right-hand page and indicates which physical system is under discussion.

Homeopathy for Cats

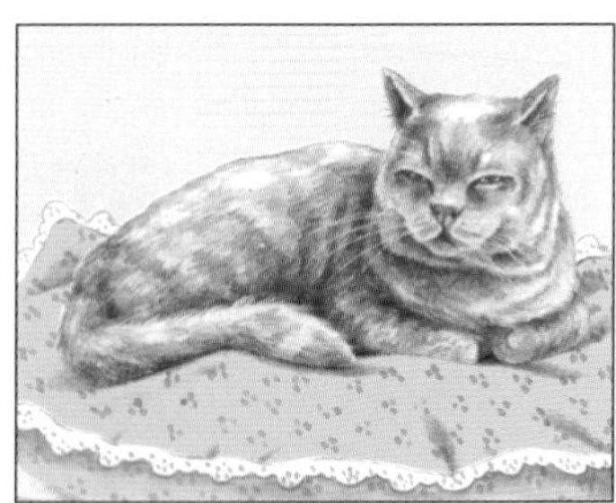

If you are fond of your cat, you will leave no stone unturned to help your pet when it is ill. At the very first symptoms of disease you need to take your cat to a veterinarian. All too frequently serious disorders are at the root of apparently innocuous symptoms. Today many veterinarians include naturopathic procedures, such as homeopathy, in their treatment arsenal.

The field of "natural" or holistic therapy, including so-called naturopathic methods, covers a broad range. It includes the use of classic homeopathic remedies and of treatment methods such as acupuncture. There now are many veterinarians who use naturopathic procedures with good success. The decision as to whether conventional medications are preferable in a particular case, however, is better left to your veterinarian.

Limits of naturopathic procedures: As a rule natural therapeutic methods are no substitute if surgery is called for, nor can they counterbalance an acute deficiency such as a calcium deficiency.

With many diseases, however, the best path of treatment surely is the one that lies between the two extremes, that is, conventional classical medicine supplemented by naturopathic procedures. Homeopathy is especially appropriate when the self-healing processes of the body need to be stimulated, but it is also helpful with metabolic or hormonal disorders.

Fever, coughing, and diarrhea often are the body's natural defense mechanisms or detoxification processes, which should not be merely suppressed.

Here, homeopathic medications have solely a regulating effect. Nevertheless, you cannot expect naturopathic procedures to produce miracle cures, although they often prove helpful even when no more headway can be made with the conventional therapeutic measures of classical medicine. They take hold, however, only if the body's processes of self-healing are still capable of being stimulated. A damaged cell may perhaps recover, but a destroyed one no longer can.

Cat owners need to realize that natural therapy as a rule takes longer than "normal" treatment with an antibiotic, for example. After all, the body first has to be stimulated to produce a reaction.

If cat owners with little experience in this field wish to treat their pets with homeopathic remedies or other naturopathic methods, we recommend that they look at their efforts only as first aid, so to speak, and undertake them only where minor illnesses are concerned or as an accompanying therapy. A serious disease may lie behind what at first glance appears to be only a minor upset. If no appreciable improvement is evident within 24 hours at most after the treatment you implement, you need to take your cat to a veterinarian in order to get at the underlying cause.

What Is Homeopathy?

Samuel Hahnemann (1755–1843), a physician, was the founder of homeopathy, which is based on the principle *Simile similibus curentur* ("Like is cured by like"). That means that where certain diseases are concerned, certain substances, diluted by potentiation, induce self-healing in the body. Undiluted, on the other hand, they cause an outbreak of precisely the same disease.

For example, after a bee sting, the bee poison produces a reddened, hot, painful swelling. If similar symptoms appear, either after an insect bite or for other reasons, you can use the venom of the honeybee (*Apis*) in diluted form to cause the symptoms to abate.

Homeopathy was an appealing alternative to the rough-and-ready medical treatments of Hahnemann's time. Thus, homeopathy became popular in Europe and was introduced to the United States in the 1820s. Its apparent successes during cholera epidemics on both continents attracted additional converts from orthodox medicine.

The initial criticisms of homeopathy in this country were prompted by professional jealousy more than anything else. Most conventional physicians did not welcome the competition from homeopaths. The American Medical Association, formed in 1847, was, in part, an attempt by orthodox physicians to vanquish their rivals. Nevertheless, by 1900, there were 22 homeopathic medical schools, more than 100 hospitals, and roughly 15,000 practitioners in the United States.

The next two decades provided the weapons that traditional physicians had been seeking in their war on homeopathy. As conventional medicine developed effective drugs and therapies and as training programs for physicians became standardized, homeopathy fell into decline. By the 1920s most American homeopathic schools had closed, and there were only a few hundred homeopathic practitioners in this country. Not until the 1970s, when Americans became enamored with natural foods and natural fibers did natural remedies return to some favor. Today, homeopathic remedies promising relief from chronic ills—allergies, arthritis, premenstrual syndrome—can even be found in chain stores.

Preparation

Vegetable (for example, *Arnica*), animal (for example, *Lachesis*), and chemical (for example, sulfur) substances, as well as products of disease (so-called nosodes), are used in the preparation of homeopathic remedies. Particularly with chronic disorders, the cat's blood or urine also can be potentized.

Potentization is the term used for the dilution and agitation or trituration (rubbing) of a substance, carried out by degrees. According to the prin-

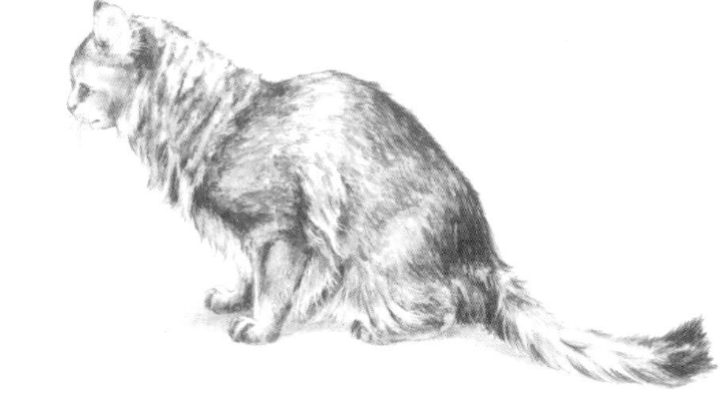

This cat doesn't feel well. That message is conveyed by its overall posture. Its coat is dull, and the cat seems apathetic.

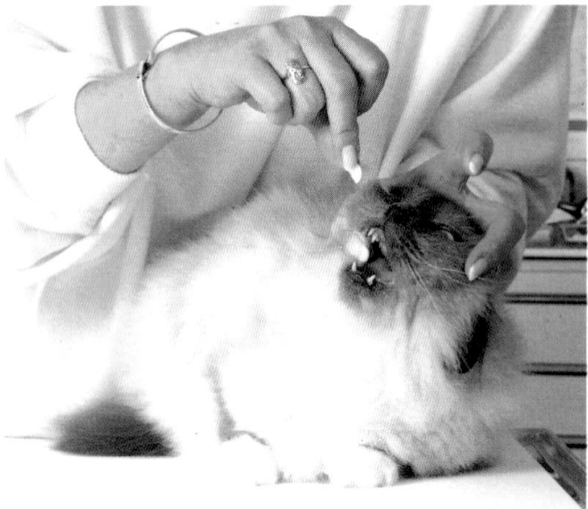

Open the cat's mouth with one hand. Lay the tablet on the back of the tongue.

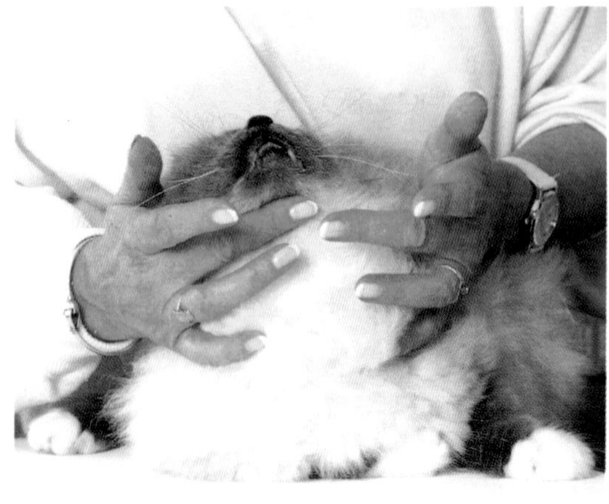

Hold the cat's mouth closed and massage its throat with your fingers until the cat swallows.

Available Forms and Dosage

Homeopathic remedies are available commercially in a variety of forms:

- drops
- tablets
- globules (sugar-coated pearls or spherules)
- powders
- ointments
- suppositories
- ampules for injection

In a single dose a cat is given:

- five to ten drops
- one tablet
- five globules
- one pinch of powder
- injections are given by a veterinarian

Overdosing is not possible as a rule and also not necessary—that is, ten tablets will not have an effect different from that of one tablet. The frequency of the treatments, however, is important. With acute conditions the remedy is administered frequently, three to six times daily. As "stoss-therapy"—massive dose therapy—it is administered with even greater frequency. In chronic cases treatments are given less often—one to three times daily, perhaps only once a week or even less frequently with very high potencies. You can work from the idea that it is not necessary to keep giving your cat a remedy as long as improvement continues. Homeopathic remedies begin to act as soon as they contact the mucous membranes in the mouth; for that reason, they should be given undiluted.

Administering homeopathic remedies to cats usually is not difficult. As a rule they take the remedies quite willingly. Frequently there are problems with drops containing alcohol. In such instances it sometimes is helpful to dilute the drops with a little water or cream. If the cat still refuses to take them, the veterinarian can inject the contents of an ampule (without alcohol) instead.

ciple of similarity, the substance that is potentized in this way will cure symptoms of disease. In concentrated form, however, it would trigger those same symptoms. This effect has not yet been explained with traditional methods. We assume that during agitation information from the substance is transferred to the solvent (diluent).

In potentization one part of a substance is diluted with nine parts of a solvent (for example, a mixture of water and ethyl alcohol) and is then agitated vigorously. This first degree of potentization, which contains the initial substance in a 1:10 ratio with water, is known as D1 (D = decimal potency or 10 potency; 1 = first degree of potentization).

If you next agitate one part of the D1 mixture with nine parts of the solvent, the initial substance is present in a 1:100 ratio. If D2 is diluted with solvent, the result is the D3 degree of potentization, and so forth.

Choosing the Potency

Low potencies—up to about D10—generally are used with acute diseases, while higher potencies tend to be used more for treatment of chronic disorders.

The effect of different potencies of the same homeopathic remedy can vary somewhat. For example, one potency may be more effective in treating diarrhea, while another works better with constipation.

If you have little experience with homeopathic remedies, you should choose potencies in the D6 to D12 range. If you use several remedies simultaneously, they should have the same potency, if at all possible.

The Right Medication

In choosing the appropriate homeopathic medication, we are guided primarily by the typical or unusual symptoms that the cat presents. General symptoms of illness such as fatigue or lack of appetite are of lesser significance. We also take into account the cat's current state of mind, temperament, and behavior. Finally, the agents that cause a disease (for example, shock or drafty air) and the circumstances under which symptoms improve or worsen (for example, factors such as warmth, cold, exercise, certain types of cat food) play a large role in our selection of the right homeopathic medication.

Close observation of the sick cat is important. Here the pet owner can contribute by providing a detailed account and ongoing reports of changes in the symptoms during treatment. Any prolonged deterioration in the cat's condition should always be reported to the veterinarian at once.

As a rule no harm is done if you have chosen the wrong remedies as long as you notify the vet if you do not see improvement within 24 hours. If you have chosen the right ones, the symptoms may become worse for a short time, but gradually the condition will improve.

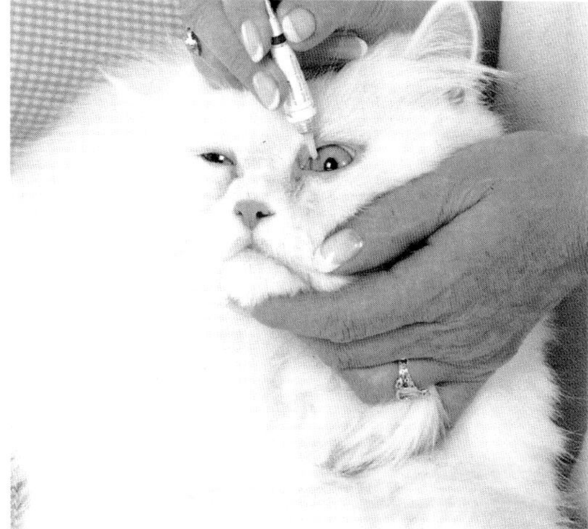

Applying eye ointment: Put one hand under the cat's chin to hold it still.

Buying and Storing Remedies

Homeopathic individual remedies and complex preparations are available in health food stores. Alternatively, veterinarians who work with these medications will provide them to you for further treatment of your cat. These medications have a very long shelf life if stored in a dry, not overly warm place.

Common Remedies

It is often difficult to describe homeopathic remedies without omitting many things of importance. If you want to learn more about the use of homeopathic medications, you need to acquire specialized literature on the subject (see "Information," page 126). I have tried to list, along with some key symptoms of each disease, those symptoms in particular that cat owners can observe fairly commonly in their pets—for example, fever, inflammations, or digestive upsets.

Apis

Apis is used with symptoms that resemble those of an insect bite. The skin or mucous membranes swell suddenly, and the affected areas are hot and painful.

A different area of application is accumulations of water in tissue (edema, see "Glossary," page 113).

Heat makes the symptoms worse.

Arnica

Arnica is helpful in treating injuries of all types (accidents, operations, wounds, bleeding, swelling, strains, shock). However, it also makes the cat react with pain when touched.

Arnica also brings relief after overexertion.

Arsenicum album

Arsenicum album is well suited for treatment of chronic disorders whose typical symptoms are lethargy, weight loss, and great thirst, although only small quantities are drunk each time. The cat has an aversion for its food, and it also vomits up food and water. If diarrhea occurs, it is eliminated in small quantities and has an unpleasant smell. The skin is usually dry and scaly.

Belladonna

Belladonna is most effective at the height of an inflammation. The symptoms appear suddenly with all the signs of inflammation, including redness and swelling, and the affected areas of skin are hot and painful. The cat's pupils are wide, and its mucous membranes are reddened and usually dry. The cat is restless and hypersensitive.

Calcium carbonicum

Calcium carbonicum is often used with young cats that suffer from swollen glands and chronic catarrhs. Their vomitus and stool have a sour smell. They cannot tolerate milk.

The preparation also helps build bone.

Hepar sulfuris

Hepar sulfuris is helpful with acute inflammations that have a tendency to fester; the altered areas are very painful. The pus is yellow and viscous.

Hepar sulfuris promotes the resolution of the suppuration.

Ipecacuanha

Ipecacuanha is very effective if the cat throws up on an empty stomach or throws up undigested food immediately after eating. The vomitus is yellow, watery, and foamy. Coughing often leads to vomiting. If bleeding occurs, the blood is light red.

Lachesis

Lachesis is used quite often with cats that are suffering from infections. The mucous membranes tend to be pallid. The animals feel worse in the morning. They dislike being touched, especially in the neck area. Solid food is easier for them to swallow than is liquid nourishment. If bleeding occurs, the blood is dark.

Lycopodium

Lycopodium is used with liver and kidney problems. Ravenous hunger is typical, but the animals are full after only a few bites. Attacks of colic and flatulence occur. The feces and urine smell unpleasant.

Club moss can also be of use with problems in the head area. The cat has trouble swallowing, and its nose is stopped with yellowish green pus. The symptoms worsen in the evenings.

Mercurius solubilis

Mercurius solubilis is effective against inflammations involving severe swelling and a tendency to hemorrhage, especially where the mucous membranes are concerned. If you apply light pressure to the cat's gums and they begin to bleed, that is evidence of a bleeding tendency.

All secretions are mucopurulent and bloody. The gums are swollen, and ulcers may form on the tongue. The animal drools and has very bad breath. If it has diarrhea, the feces is blood tinged and mucid, and the anus is sore.

Natrium muriaticum

Natrium muriaticum, or common salt, is used when a cat is losing weight although it has a good appetite and when it has a strong craving for salt. The animal's sudden mood change is striking. Eczema appears, accompanied by itching, pustules, and scaliness.

Nux vomica

Nux vomica is useful for treating the consequences of eating too much food, the wrong food, or spoiled food. If colic results, the animal arches its back. Frequently, the cat has severe constipation; it strains, but without success. Vomiting often occurs in the mornings. Some cats have bouts of ravenous hunger. Many cats are nervous and irritable.

Phosphorus

Phosphorus is used for a cat that tires quickly but also recovers quickly. The cat is highly sensitive to noise and has a strong tendency to hemorrhage. It is thirsty for cold water, which it vomits up after drinking.

Pulsatilla

Pulsatilla is used to treat suppurations with thick, creamy, yellowish green secretions. The state of the cat's stool changes. Problems appear especially after the cat has eaten fat. The animal dislikes being in a warm room.

Rhus toxicodendron

Rhus toxicodendron is used with illnesses resulting from cold and wet weather and after overexertion (muscles, tendons). These symptoms can often be observed with colds: sneezing, conjunctivitis accompanied by an aversion to light, difficulty swallowing, and dry coughing. After overexertion the cat's legs are stiff when it stands up, but after plenty of exercise it becomes more limber again.

Silicea

Silicea is used to promote complete healing of suppurations of all kinds, fistulas, and wounds. The secretions have an unpleasant smell. The cat has an aversion to meat; milk is tolerated poorly.

Sulfur

Sulfur is an important reagent with chronic illnesses or poor healing (give one D30 dose of sulfur). The animals' coats are rough, unclean, shaggy, and smelly. Diarrhea and constipation alternate; the body orifices are reddened.

▪ Homeopathy to Treat Infections

Fever is one of several attendant symptoms in a wide variety of diseases. For this reason we present the following homeopathic remedies that are applicable with all diseases accompanied by fever. Please note also the homeopathy tips appearing in the individual chapters of the disease section.

For dosages, see page 60.

Fever

- Acute fever, sudden pain, restlessness, reddened mucous membranes, dilated pupils, fever without thirst: *Belladonna*.
- Acute course of illness, high fever, mucous membranes rather pallid, pain in neck area, worse in the mornings: *Lachesis*.
- Moderate, persistent fever or recurring fever: *Ferrum phosphoricum*.
- Beginnings of infection or suppuration; to increase resistance: *Echinacea*.

1

Disorders of the Head Area

In a life spent in the wild a cat's keen eyes and sensitive hearing are vital to its survival. Only with their help can the cat stalk and catch a mouse even in the densest tangle of plant growth. To kill its prey and break it up into smaller pieces, the cat uses its sharp, fanged teeth.

Diseases of the eyes, ears, or teeth, therefore, can seriously interfere with the cat's natural way of life.

Conjunctivitis

Symptoms: Tearing eyes (see photo below), watery and clear to mucopurulent flow of tears, aversion to light, spasmodic closing of lid, reddening and swelling of conjunctiva.

Causes: Foreign body in eye (speck of dust, sand), allergies. Rarely, congenital malformation of lid and hairs that cause irritation. In most cases infection-causing agents trigger conjunctivitis. Some viruses, chlamydia (see "Glossary," page 113), and bacteria are the primary agents. Other bacteria colonize secondarily once an inflammation is present. Often the disease is an attendant symptom of the feline respiratory disease complex (see page 107) in which primarily herpes viruses cause serious harm.

Chlamydia can be transmitted to unborn kittens while still in their mother's body. Then the little kittens often are born with a serious eye infection, present even before their eyelids open on about the ninth day.

Effects: The disease also can spread to the sclera (see "Glossary," page 113) and cornea.

● Treatment

For irritation of the conjunctiva with a watery and clear or mucopurulent flow of tears, clean the rims of the eyelids two or three times a day, using a soft paper tissue dipped in lukewarm water or in a chamomile solution (see "How-to: "Preventive Care," page 14).

▶ A clinical examination is necessary to tell whether an infection is present or whether other causes have to be considered. Above all it is important to detect a systemic infection when the conjunctivitis is

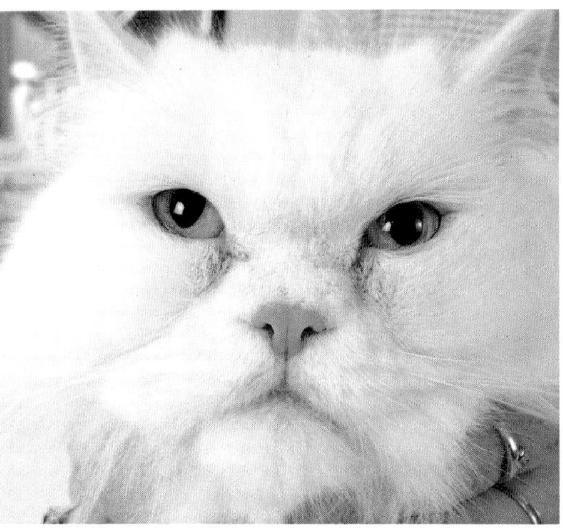

Many Persians tend to have a constant flow of tears. This is not always a symptom of disease, therefore.

only one of the symptoms. In many cases therapy entails the use of eye drops or ointments that contain antibiotics.

Injections of antibiotics are the most likely to succeed with the commonly occurring chlamydia infection. In intractable cases taking a swab from the cornea can provide more information. If the conjunctivitis is due to a malformation of the eyelid, surgery is necessary.

Follow-up care: Apply eye drops four to six times a day or eye ointment two or three times a day for one week (see "Nursing a Sick Cat," page 50). Regularly clean of the rims of the eyelids, which are stuck together with secretions.

Prevention: Prevent drafts (for example, through open windows and doors), and don't let the cat's head get extremely dirty.

Susceptible breeds: Persian cats, with their big eyes, tight conjunctival sac, and short, flattened noses, often have a constant trickle of tears without any signs of conjunctivitis.

Try not to use severely affected animals for breeding purposes.

■ **Homeopathy**

See page 67.

Irises of Different Colors

Symptoms: Eyes of different colors—for example, one light yellow iris and one orange iris. An unpigmented (light blue) iris can appear in one eye.

Causes: Hereditary predisposition. In albino cats (see "Glossary," page 113) and in Siamese and other masked cats, the blue iris color is caused by lack of pigment (hypochromia).

A purebred cat with a white coat and light blue irises may be congenitally deaf.

● **Treatment**

No treatment possible.

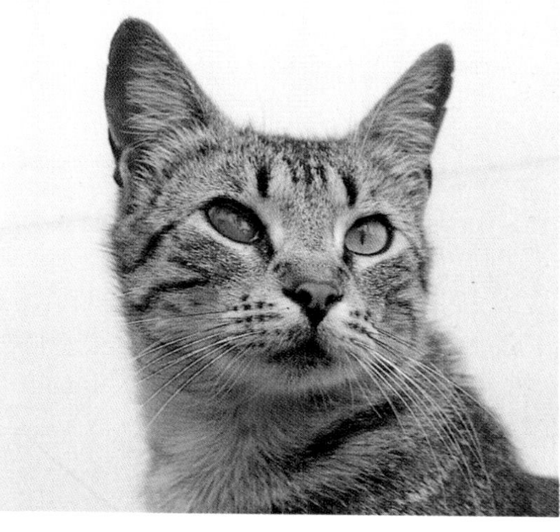

The cloudiness of the cornea of this cat's right eye can be a result of inflammatory processes or injuries (see below).

Prevention: Do not breed cats with hereditary disorders.

Diseases of the Eyeball

Symptoms: Shrinkage, absence, or atrophy of the eyeball.

Causes: Genetic trait, inflammation, injuries. When bruises occur (accidents, fights), blood can enter the chamber of the eye and cause injuries inside the eye. After severe skull injuries the entire eyeball can protrude from the socket.

● **Treatment**

▶ Possible only by a veterinarian. In addition to treatment with antibiotics, surgical measures are often necessary.

Follow-up care: Ointments and drops containing antibiotics usually are given over a fairly long period of time.

Inflammation of the Cornea (Keratitis)

Symptoms: Spasmodic closing of lid, flow of tears, gray film, opacity; if course of disease is protracted and severe, blood vessels will develop on the cornea.

Causes: Injuries caused by claws, blows, or foreign bodies are starting points for the inflammation; infections.

Effects: Inflammation of the cornea (keratitis) frequently goes hand in hand with conjunctivitis. If the disease takes an unfavorable course, a corneal ulcer is often the result. If the ulcer breaks through the cornea, the aqueous fluid can leak out, leading to loss of the eye.

● **Treatment**

▶ Possible only by a veterinarian. With infections or injuries broad-spectrum antibiotics are used (see "Glossary," page 113). In special cases a protective covering is made (contact lenses or third eyelid-conjunctival flaps).

Follow-up care: Administer eye drops and ointment several times a day, depending on the severity of the case, until the eye is completely healed.

Susceptible breeds: A congenital malformation of the cornea (corneal dystrophy) occurs in Manx cats.

■ **Homeopathy**

See page 67.

Protrusion of the Nictitating Membrane

Symptoms: The nictitating membrane (third eyelid) is pushed up from the lower lid and the corner of the nose and is visible over the corner of the eyeball as a whitish-pink membrane.

Causes: Many general diseases, including severe parasite infestation (see "Disorders Caused by Parasites," page 96). If the eyeball has too much or too little room in its socket—for example, as a result of dehydration, wasting diseases, or swelling—the nictitating membrane frequently becomes visible.

● **Treatment**

▶ Possible only by the veterinarian. The therapy depends on the underlying disease.

Follow-up care: In many cases treatment with eye drops prescribed by the veterinarian. Apply eye ointment four to six times daily.

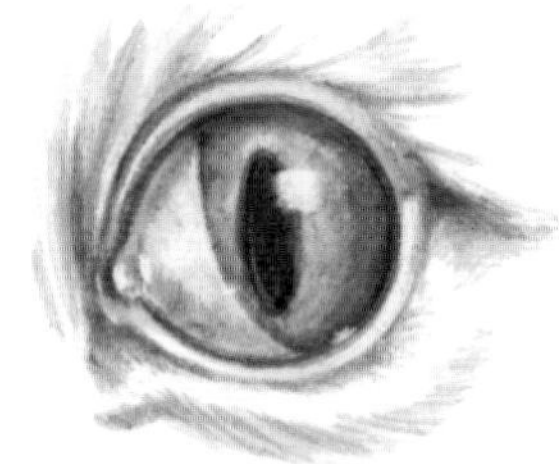

Prolapse of the nictitating membrane is a symptom of a variety of diseases.

Glaucoma

Symptoms: Bulging, enlarged globe with fixed pupil through which the back of the retina shows with a green glow; nebula; lens change.

Causes: If the internal pressure in the eyeball continues to rise as a result of increased aqueous humor, we use the term glaucoma. Glaucoma can develop in the eyeball without any external cause or after injuries, inflammations, and tumors.

● **Treatment**

▶ Possible only by the veterinarian. In the initial stage diuretic medications (see "Glossary," page 113) are used to lower the intraocular pressure. Only surgery, which the veterinarian can perform, can bring permanent help.

Change in the Lens

Symptoms: Milky-white opacity of the lens.

Causes: Genetic trait, injuries, infections, sign of degeneration in advanced age.

Effects: Range from weak sight to blindness.

● **Treatment**

▶ Possible only by the veterinarian. In many cases veterinary surgery will preserve the cat's strength of vision.

■ Homeopathy with Eye Disorders

For dosages, see page 60.

- Swollen lids: *Apis, Arsenicum album, Causticum, Hepar sulfuris, Rhus toxicodendron.*
- Swollen lids, spasmodically closed: *Mercurius solubilis.*
- Flow of tears: *Cepa, Euphrasia.*
- Conjunctivitis: *Arsenicum album, Calcium carbonicum, Causticum, Hepar sulfuris, Ipecacuanha, Rhus toxicodendron,* sulfur.

Nystagmus

Symptoms: Jerking movements of the eyeballs.

Causes: Hereditary predisposition; brain damage resulting from injuries or from infections of the central nervous system.

● Treatment

No treatment possible with hereditary predisposition.

▶ If the eye tremor is an accompanying symptom of brain damage, the veterinarian has to search for the cause. Successful treatment is possible in only a few cases. The prognosis is usually guarded or grave.

Diseases of the Retina

Symptoms: Range from weak vision to blindness.

Causes: Progressive degeneration of the retina, which is hereditary (feline progressive retinal atrophy, PRA); hemorrhages, retinal degeneration, and inflammation can be associated with infections; retinal diseases caused by nutritional deficiency—e.g., lack of taurine (see page 21).

● Treatment

▶ Possible only by the veterinarian. The fundus oculi (back of the eye) is viewed through the lens with a special lamp (ophthalmoscope; see "Glossary," page 113).

- If the retinal disease is caused by an infection, the underlying disease first has to be identified. It will determine the therapy.
- Nutritionally caused retinal diseases can be remedied by a diet of foods with high nutritional value (see page 16).
- PRA is incurable.

Follow-up care: Administer medications as directed by the veterinarian.

Prevention: Do not use animals with PRA for breeding purposes. Make sure your cat's diet is adequate.

Susceptible breeds: PRA has been found in Persians, Siamese, and Abyssinians.

External Ear Injury

Symptoms: Wounds; deformation of the external ear.

Causes: Lacerations and bites received in fights, congenital deformity.

Effects: Festering inflammation, hematoma.

● Treatment

Small wounds and scratches heal on their own.

▶ Larger wounds and festering inflammations need the attention of a veterinarian. A hematoma can assume such proportions that it has to be removed surgically.

Follow-up care: Apply antibiotic ointment two or three times a day.

Susceptible breeds: In Scottish fold cats, a congenital mutation of the external ear appears.

■ Homeopathy

See page 73.

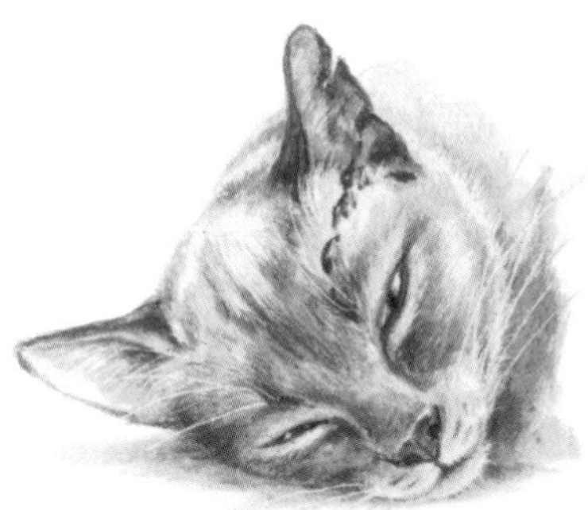

Bite marks on the external ear.

Inflammations of the Outer Auditory Canal

Symptoms: The cat scratches and paws at its ear, shakes its head, and holds it at an angle. There are dirty, brown secretions in the ear canal.

Causes: Ear mites (see "Disorders Caused by Parasites," page 96), foreign bodies, bacteria, and fungi cause infections that usually appear in the course of ear mite infestation.

Effects: Festering skin inflammations and abscesses can be caused by the cat's scratching.

● **Treatment**

▶ The veterinarian will look at the ear canal with a special instrument (otoscope, see "Glossary," page 113, and photo, page 48). Ear mites have to be detected with a microscope.

• Treatment of ear mites (see page 96).

• Foreign bodies in the ear are removed by the veterinarian.

The auditory canal is thoroughly cleaned with an ear-cleaning solution and a cotton-tipped applicator, followed by treatment with antibiotic ointment. With rare, treatment-resistant forms of bacteria and fungi, additional tests have to be made.

Follow-up care: See "Ear Mites," page 96. Weekly check-up by the veterinarian until healing is complete.

Prevention: Regular inspection of the ears.

■ **Homeopathy**
See page 78.

Infection of the Middle Ear

Symptoms: General condition is impaired, cat tilts its head down on the affected side. Equilibrium can be disturbed if the inner ear is also involved.

Causes: A serious, improperly treated infection of the auditory canal (*otitis externa*) can, if the eardrum is destroyed, lead to an infection of the middle ear (*otitis media*). It is also possible for the middle ear to become infected as a result of an inflammation in the head cavity.

Effects: Sometimes a severe middle ear infection also affects the inner ear.

● **Treatment**

▶ Possible only by the veterinarian. In addition to a thorough cleaning of the auditory canal with ear-cleaning solution and a cotton-tipped applicator, injections of antibiotics are given.

As a rule eardrum injuries heal quite well.

Follow-up care: Check ears regularly, and administer ointments or drops as the veterinarian directs.

■ Homeopathy with Mouth and Throat Disorders

For dosages, see page 60.

• Blisters, ulcers: *Lycopodium*, sulfur, *Thuja, Mercurius solubilis, Apis, Lac caninum.*

• Red border along edge of gums: *Natrium nitricum, Mercurius solubilis.*

• Pain upon opening mouth: *Argentum nitricum.*

• Heavy drooling: *Mercurius solubilis, Natrium muriaticum, Phytolacca.*

• Dry mucous membranes: *Belladonna, Cimifuga, Carbo vegetabilis.*

Plaque and Tartar

Symptoms: Dense, brownish gray deposit on the teeth, sometimes bad breath. Staining substances (for example, Natrium-Fluorescin) can reveal the deposit.

Tartar is easy to detect when you inspect the cat's oral cavity (see photo, page 69). Tartar is usually heaviest on the outer side of the large molars.

Causes: The surface of the teeth is colonized by microbes. They form a deposit and attack the dental substance. After a certain time these deposits calcify and turn into tartar, which continues to spread.

Effects: Inflammation of the gums, formation of periodontal pockets, gum proliferations, suppuration of the dental roots.

● **Treatment**

▶ Tartar is removed by the veterinarian, either mechanically or with ultrasound under anesthesia. Topical disinfection and treatment before and after with antibiotics increase the likelihood of successful treatment.

Follow-up care: For healing and prevention disinfect teeth and edges of gums with a 2 percent solution of hydrogen peroxide at least twice a week (apply with a cotton swab). Many cats, however, object to such treatment. It is also possible to control the deposits with antibiotics. The dose is calculated by a veterinarian on the basis of the cat's body weight.

Prevention: Hard, dry cat food and raw, gristly foods, along with natural prey, have a cleansing function.

Regular brushing with a miniature toothbrush or a pet toothpaste may be useful for some cats, though not all cats will allow this treatment.

■ **Homeopathy**

See page 68.

Inflammation of the Gums (Gingivitis)

Symptoms: Tartar, inflammation at the edge of the gums, difficulty eating, drooling, bad breath.

Causes: Production of harmful substances by tartar.

Effects: Dense clumps of tartar, periodontal pockets, loosening and festering of individual teeth.

● **Treatment**

▶ The veterinarian will remove the tartar deposits with the cat placed under anesthesia. Gum proliferation and periodontal pockets are treated surgically, and loose and damaged teeth are pulled; treatment with antibiotics.

Follow-up care: Give antibiotics for about one week.

Prevention: See "Plaque and Tartar," page 68.

■ **Homeopathy**

See page 68.

Malocclusions

Irregularities of tooth formation are inherited. In "true-to-type" Persian cats in particular, these irregularities appear in the form of an overly short (undershot) upper jaw. More rarely, an overly long (overshot) upper jaw and an overly short, weak lower jaw are seen in long-headed, slender forms of cats (Siamese, for example). Cats with pronounced malocclusions should not be used for breeding.

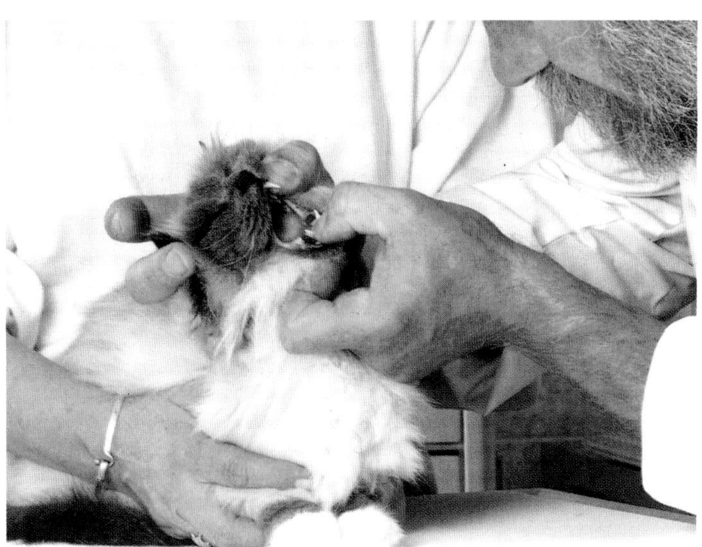

The veterinarian is checking this cat's teeth.

Disorders of the Locomotor and Nervous Systems

The skeleton protects sensitive organs from external injury and gives the cat its overall structure. The rigid skeletal system is moved by means of the joints. Closely linked with the locomotor apparatus is the nervous system, which extends through the entire body. The brain, in combination with the spinal cord, constitutes the central nervous system.

Osteoporosis

Symptoms: Osteoporosis affects young animals almost exclusively. They look weak and undernourished.

Causes: Malnutrition; chronic inflammation of the bowels because of severe worm infestation (see page 127). A hereditary predisposition appears to be present in some cat breeds.

Effects: Skeletal deformation, stunted growth, bone breakage.

- **Treatment**

▶ The veterinarian will recommend a diet of high nutritive value, rich in protein (see "Proper Nutrition," page 16). Worm-infested cats have to be dewormed (see "Deworming Schedule," page 27).

Follow-up care and prevention: See "Proper Nutrition," page 16.

Conservative Treatment or Orthopedic Surgery?

By "conservative treatment" we mean all procedures that promote healing, for example, bandages, splints, and plaster casts. Orthopedic surgery is not performed.

Modern veterinary orthopedic surgery is conversant with techniques such as inserting a metal pin, bolting or screwing bones into position, stabilizing bones with metal plates, resectioning (removing troublesome fragments), and inserting artificial parts.

Advantages and disadvantages are involved in both methods of treatment. Conservative treatment continues to be appropriate with quite a few of the cat's fractures, including pelvic fractures, many fractures of the femur and humerus, and fractures of the shoulder blade and ribs. They heal nicely.

With certain injuries forgoing surgical repair can potentially result in improper healing. The consequences include shortening, ankylosis or abnormal positioning of limbs, development of false articulations, and permanent joint damage.

Hint: With both treatment methods you always need to keep in mind that cats may have a hypersensitive reaction to fixed dressings after pinning or similar procedures, to Elizabethan collars (to keep the cat from licking and nibbling at the wound), and especially to being locked in a pet hospital cage. They sometimes lapse into a depressive state and refuse to eat.

Joint Dysplasia

Symptoms: If a severe abnormality is present, the cat is lame.

Causes and effects: By dysplasia we mean the congenital or acquired malformation of a joint in which the articular facets (surfaces) do not fit precisely on top of one another. Hereditary dysplasia can take a great variety of forms, influenced by different factors (nutrition, strain). Changes in joints can also develop as a result of injuries and of favoring the joint because of pain. Hip dysplasia (HD) in dogs is of particular importance. HD also appears in cats, but is of less significance for them because their way of life is affected only by severe forms of HD.

Luxation (see "Glossary," page 113) of the kneecap and cartilage damage are also inherited problems.

● **Treatment**

▶ Diagnosis can be made only by x-ray. As a rule affected cats do not need treatment. In severe cases surgery can help.

Prevention: In purebred cats hereditary dysplasia must be prevented by selective breeding.

Disorders of the Locomotor Apparatus

Symptoms: Lameness, tenderness, swelling, unnatural positions, or abnormal flexibility of the affected limb.

Causes: Injuries in accidents; the joints are sprained, usually with tears in the articular capsule; tendons and ligaments are torn; separation of the connections to muscles and nerves; fractures.

● **Treatment**

▶ In many cases the veterinarian can make a diagnosis by examination and palpation (see "Glossary," page 113) of the animal and by observation of the cat's behavior. Radiographs provide information on the nature and location of fractures and dislocations. The cat is anesthetized before being radiographed.

In some cases surgery can bring relief (see "Conservative Treatment or Orthopedic Surgery?" page 70). The veterinarian will either perform the surgery or refer the cat to an orthopedic veterinary surgeon.

■ **Homeopathy**

See page 73.

Vitamin A Poisoning

Symptoms: Pain when cat moves, reluctance to move.

Causes: Excessive amounts of Vitamin A in food (see page 22).

Effects: In the course of the poisoning (hypervitaminosis A) joint damage, abnormal ossification, and ankylosis of joints can occur.

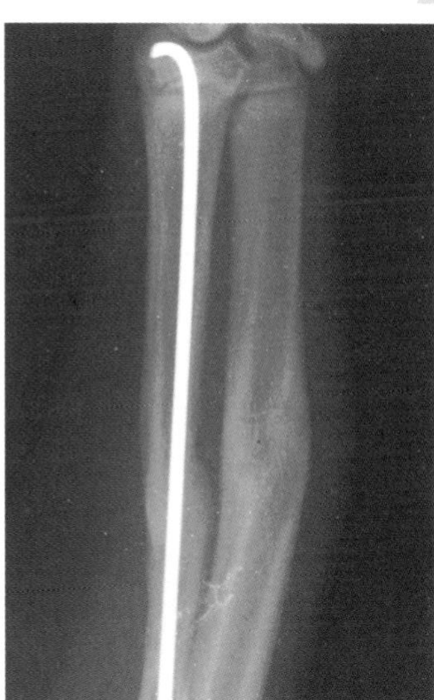

Radiograph of a pinning of a long bone that was fractured.

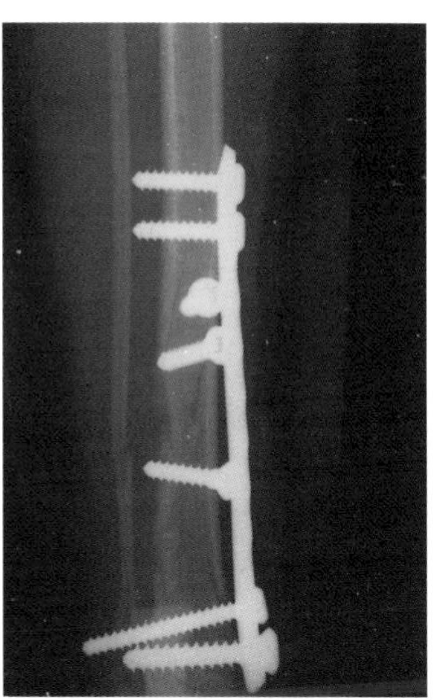

A metal plate stabilizes the fractured long bone.

● **Treatment**

▶ Diagnosis is made by the veterinarian. Radiographs provide information on the level of joint damage.

Nutritional counseling by the veterinarian.

Follow-up care and prevention: Avoid excess of Vitamin A in food (see "Nutritional Disorders," page 20). A chief cause of Vitamin A poisoning is overly frequent servings of liver.

Inflammation of Joints

A joint is a movable link between two bones. The two smooth articular facets, which fit together precisely, glide past one another with friction being diminished by synovial fluid. The fibrous articular capsule stabilizes the joint and separates it from the surrounding tissue. If one or more of these functional parts is subjected to changes, an inflammation of the joint arises. For acute processes we use the term arthritis, for chronic processes, arthrosis.

Symptoms: Pain when the cat moves: it tries to favor the affected joint. It limps more or less conspicuously.

Causes: Bruises or strains, infections.

● **Treatment**

▶ Possible only by the veterinarian. The joint actually ought to be immobilized, but cats favor it of their own accord. Heat can promote healing.

With infections or processes where there is a risk of infection (for example, a bite wound in the joint), treatment with antibiotics has to be administered, generally by injection.

Follow-up care: Injections of antibiotics by the veterinarian. Help the healing process along by arranging a warm, dry bed for the cat to lie on (see illustration, page 51). Let your pet get plenty of rest, and provide water, food, and a litter box nearby.

■ **Homeopathy**

See page 73.

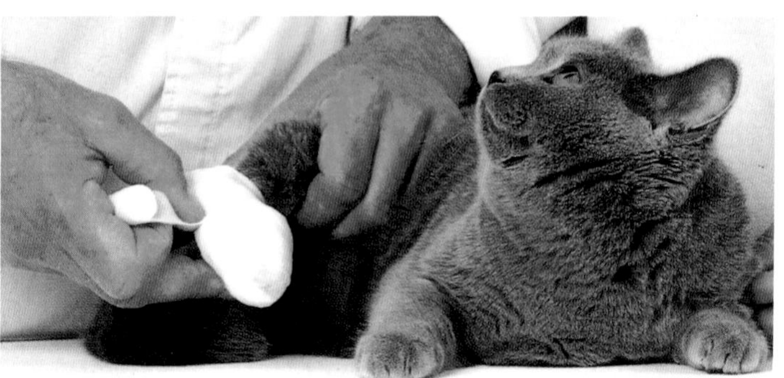

Cats often are quick to tear off dressings.

Infections of the Central Nervous System

Symptoms: Changes in behavior (for example, drowsiness, trembling, compulsive movements, disturbance of equilibrium, fearfulness, or aggression).

Causes: Many feline viral infections, including rabies, affect the central nervous system and the brain (see "Infectious Diseases," page 104). Bacterial encephalitis can develop in the course of systemic infections and with suppurating diseases in the head area.

● **Treatment**

▶ Any signs of central nervous system disturbance require immediate veterinary care. Put the cat in the carrier and handle as little as possible until the veterinarian has examined the animal. The veterinarian has to determine the cause. If the brain has been attacked by viruses causing rabies, FIP, FeLV, FIV, or Aujeszky's disease (see "Infectious Diseases," page 104), no therapy can bring about a cure. The cat should be put to sleep (see "Euthanasia," page 45).

Homeopathy with Wounds and Injuries

For dosages, see page 60.
- Acute injuries of all kinds, hemorrhage, swelling, shock: *Arnica.*
- Consequences of overexertion: *Arnica.*
- Fresh and infected wounds: *Calendula.*
- Injuries of the ligaments and tendons: *Rhus toxicodendron.*
- Bone injuries: *Symphytum.*
- Slow-healing wounds, excessive scar formation: *Silicea.*
- Acute reddening, heat, pain: *Hepar sulfuris.*
- After the acute phase: *Myristica sebifera.*
- Hard swelling, watery, foul-smelling secretion: *Mercurius solubilis.*
- Viscous, creamy pus: *Pulsatilla.*

Sometimes bacterial infections still can be remedied by prompt use of appropriate antibiotics and corticosteroids (see "Glossary," page 113).

Follow-up care: With bacterial infections antibiotics are administered for about two weeks.

Vitamin B Deficiency

Symptoms: Disturbed behavior, head held at an angle, loss of coordination and staggering gait, seizures, blindness.

Causes: Malnutrition (see page 21), infection of the central nervous system (see page 72), concomitant of feline respiratory disease (see page 107), severe infestation with intestinal parasites (see page 100).

Effects: Over the long run Vitamin B deficiency can result in permanent brain damage.

● Treatment

▶ Have veterinarian determine causes. Besides treatment of the secondary disorder, Vitamin B injections need to be given.

Follow-up care and prevention: Administer medications as veterinarian directs. If malnutrition is present, make sure the cat's food has the proper balance of nutrients.

Brain Injuries

Symptoms: Loss of consciousness, dazed state, changes in eyes.

Causes and effects: Accidents, blows to the head; as a result, brain concussion, cerebral contusions, rupture and bleeding of the brain.

● Treatment

▶ The cat has to be taken to a veterinarian immediately. He or she will decide whether to radiograph the cat.
- With cerebral contusions and disorientation the cat usually recovers on its own. Therapy with analgesic, calming medications and B vitamins can be helpful.
- If blood vessels in the brain rupture, the extravasated blood causes pressure damage in the brain (hematoma). The veterinarian will prescribe diuretics (which promote elimination of water) in order to lower the pressure.
- Depending on the injury, surgery or treatment with antibiotics is necessary.

Follow-up care: A comfortable bed (see illustration, page 51) and peace and quiet promote the healing process. Administer diuretics and antibiotics as the veterinarian directs.

■ Homeopathy

See above.

Disorders of the Skin and the Hormonal Glands

The skin, along with the coat of hair, encloses the cat's body like a protective mantle. In addition, the skin regulates the influence of temperature factors and transmits information. A cat changes its coat in spring and in fall. When the weather gets colder outdoors, the coat becomes thicker, and in warmer temperatures it sheds hair. A multitude of nerve endings, spread throughout the skin, report to the brain information such as a sensation of pain or changes in temperature.

Alopecia (Balding)

Symptoms: Range from development of isolated bald patches to baldness extending over the entire body.

Causes: Hereditary predisposition; hormonal disorders (see page 77), abnormal behavior (constant licking), chronic skin diseases (for example, parasite infestation, fungi, allergies).

● **Treatment**

▶ The veterinarian can provide a specific diagnosis based on the manifestation and on special lab tests. Health problems such as parasite infestations, allergies, infections, or hormonal disorders have to be treated individually.

Follow-up care and prevention: Balanced diet and appropriate living conditions. Make sure the cat remains free of parasites (see page 96).

Susceptible breeds: Inherited lack of hair occurs in the hairless cat (Sphynx), but this does not mean the cat inherits the diseases of which hairlessness is a symptom.

■ **Homeopathy**

See page 78.

Abscesses

Symptoms: Hard swelling beneath the surface of the skin, later becoming softer as pus forms. If the abscess breaks through the skin, the pus drains.

Causes: Abscesses usually result from scratches and particularly from bites. For this reason they are especially common in the head and neck area and at the base of the tail.

● **Treatment**

▶ Possible only by the veterinarian, who first will administer an injection of antibiotics. If the abscess is ripe, it will be lanced. Then the wound will be disinfected.

Follow-up care: Check on the healing process regularly. You can carefully remove any crusts that interfere with the drainage of the pus, or you can ask the veterinarian to remove them.

■ **Homeopathy**

See page 78.

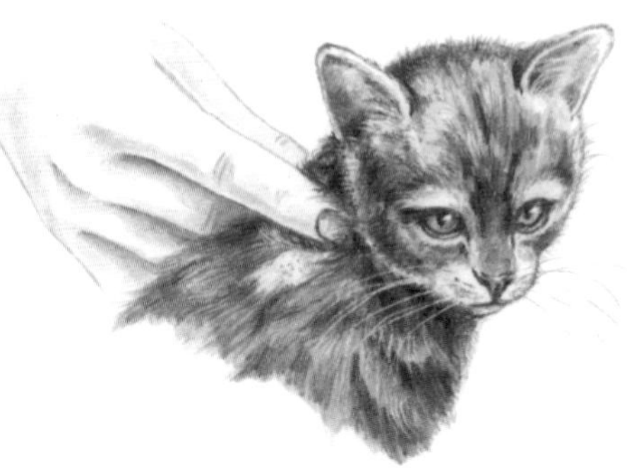

Hair loss often is evident at only one spot in the cat's coat, but it can spread quickly.

Bacterial Skin Diseases

The skin of even healthy cats is colonized by bacteria. Usually the cat is in equilibrium with these normal skin flora. Under certain circumstances, however—possibly because the animal has lowered resistance or because its skin has already suffered damage from a previous injury—a bacterial skin infection (pyoderma) can result.

Symptoms: Severe erythema; weeping eczema; purulent, crusty lesions of the skin (exudate, see "Glossary," page 113).

Causes: Scratches, grazes, and bites; becoming extremely dirty; parasite infestation; burns, including acid burns. One special form of the disease is inflammation of the nail bed.

Risk to humans: A few rare bacterial pathogens can also attack humans. In a specific case ask the veterinarian (see page 110).

● **Treatment**

▶ The veterinarian will make the exact diagnosis. He or she will take skin samples by scraping (skin scrapings, see "Glossary," page 113), and they will be examined by a microbiologist.

Many bacteria, depending on the size of the area involved, are treated with topical antibiotics for three to six weeks. Often treatment by injection is also helpful.

Follow-up care and prevention: Antibiotics as directed by veterinarian. Appropriate living conditions, balanced diet, and, above all, attention promote the healing process.

■ **Homeopathy**

See page 78.

Skin Tumors

In the skin, as in all other body tissues, cells can degenerate and tumors can form. Not all swellings are malignant, however.

● **Treatment**

▶ Examination of the tissue under a microscope (or by histopathology) will reveal whether a tumor is benign or malignant. Tumors that are detected early can be removed surgically, often with good prospects for success.

Follow-up care: Sutured incisions have to be checked daily to biweekly, depending on the progress of the healing. Nibbling or intense licking of the wound, behavior uncommon in cats, can possibly be prevented with an Elizabethan collar.

■ **Homeopathy**

Treatments with a variety of natural remedies are possible, but should be left to an experienced therapist.

Acne

Symptoms: Oily, sebaceous plugs on the chin, small pimple-like bumps, pain when touched.

Causes: Sebaceous glands and hair follicles (see "Glossary," page 113) become inflamed by impurities (mushy food).

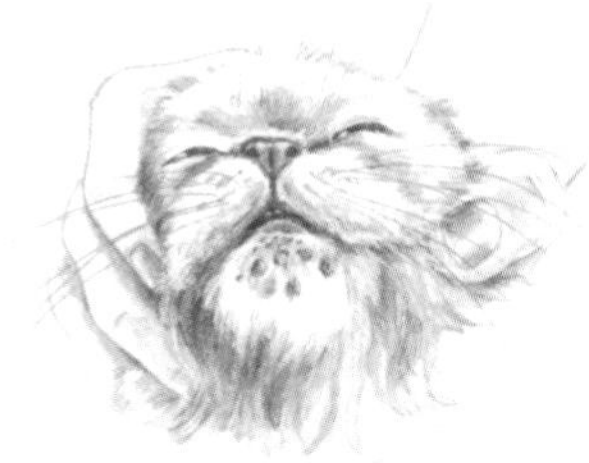

Cats get acne too.

● **Treatment**

▶ The veterinarian will clean the area with a disinfectant solution and treat it with ointment. If complications arise through formation of pus, the treatment will also include injections of antibiotics.

Follow-up care and prevention: Clean the cat's chin daily with a paper tissue dipped in a mild disinfectant solution. Ask your veterinarian for an appropriate disinfectant.

■ **Homeopathy**

See page 78.

Stud Tail

Symptoms: Oily, sebaceous plugs on the top of the tail near its base; small pimplelike bumps; the tail hairs are matted and greasy and are yellowish-brown in color.

Causes: The sebaceous glands on the upper side of the tail are secreting too much oil.

Impurities can cause the sebaceous glands and hair follicles to become inflamed.

Primarily breeding studs are affected, but females and castrated males are also candidates.

● Treatment

In mild cases wash the tail with baby shampoo, warm water, and a soft toothbrush until your hand and the cat's coat are clean.

▶ Severe cases can be treated only by a veterinarian, who will use disinfectant ointment or gel. If complications are caused by pus formation, the cat will be given injections of antibiotics.

Prevention: Once a week rub talcum powder into the hair on the tail, allow the powder to work overnight, and brush it out thoroughly the next day.

■ Homeopathy

See page 78.

Fungal Infection of the Skin

Symptoms: Isolated rounded alterations in the skin; at these places the hair becomes brittle and falls out; skin reddened and scaly; itching, often not very pronounced; with invasion of the nail bed, the matrix becomes reddened, inflamed, and swollen.

Causes: Skin fungi, or dermatophytes (see page 111). Because the spores of the fungus can stay in the environment and remain infectious for years, an infection also can be contracted without direct physical contact with diseased animals, via grooming tools, other objects, or vectors. The incubation period (see "Glossary," page 113) is at least two weeks. Some cats are carriers of dermatophytes but do not become ill themselves; they can infect other animals, however.

Risk to humans: Skin fungi are communicable to humans. For this reason try to practice scrupulous hygiene, and always wash after touching the cat with your hands (see "Important Notes," page 127)!

● Treatment

▶ The veterinarian has to find out which fungal infestation is present. Some fungi are detectable with ultraviolet light (Wood's lamp), others through inspection of the hair under a microscope. The most accurate diagnostic procedure is growing a fungus culture from skin and hair samples. Unfortunately, it takes at least one week to produce a result. To provide immediate help the veterinarian will treat the cat with an ointment or a solution that will inhibit the growth of fungi (antimycotic, see "Glossary," page 113). In addition the cat will be given tablets containing the antifungal drug Griseofulvin for at least six weeks.

If the nail bed is inflamed, the same treatment is used, but over a period of five months.

Follow-up care: Treatment of the affected portion of skin with ointment, solution, and tablets as directed by the veterinarian. The surroundings have to be disinfected (fungicide, see "Glossary," page 113).

Prevention: Optimum living conditions. When grooming your pet's coat, keep an eye out for changes in its skin.

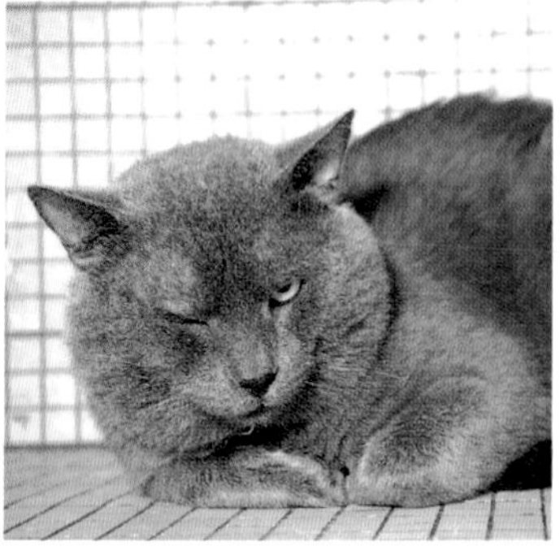

Skin diseases are common in cats.

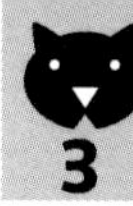

■ **Homeopathy**
See page 78.

Allergies

Symptoms: Allergies can produce an enormous variety of symptoms. For cat owners the most obvious signs to look for are intense itching, hair loss, and development of eczema.

Causes: Allergies result from misdirected defense mechanisms (antigen-antibody reaction). The following allergens (see "Glossary," page 113) are possibilities:

• Proteins in the cat's food. Food allergies sometimes appear even when the cat has been used to the food for years (see "Food Allergies," page 22).

• Flea allergies (see "Disorders Caused by Parasites," page 96).

• A genetically based allergic skin inflammation (dermatosis) is also known as atopy.

● **Treatment**

▶ Possible only by the veterinarian, who has to determine the cause. Ruling out suspected allergens can make the preliminary diagnosis firm, and the process is simultaneously the most important therapeutic procedure as well.

• With food allergies, special diets are used, first to determine the cause, then for treatment.

• With flea allergies, the parasite has to be controlled (see "Disorders Caused by Parasites," page 96).

• With allergic dermatosis, cortisone (see "Glossary," page 113) is used to alleviate the discomfort. Only after the cause has been clearly identified can it be eliminated, so that permanent healing can take place.

• In some cases allergy testing and hyposensitization injections, as are used in humans, are also helpful.

■ **Homeopathy**
See page 78.

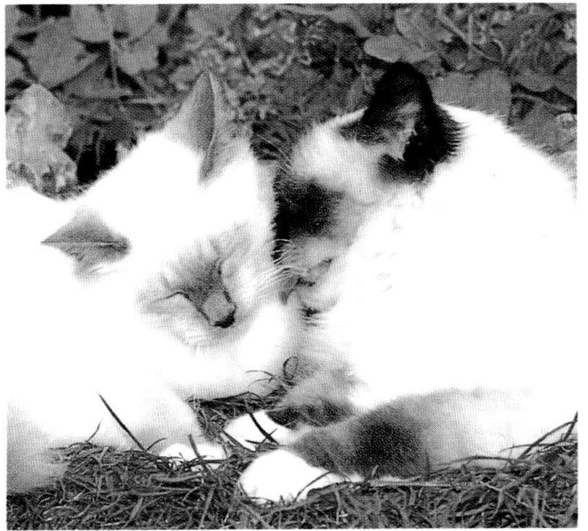

One cat tenderly licks the other's coat. These two cats are fond of one another.

Hormone-induced Disorders

Here only those hormonal problems that are most common and whose symptoms are relatively easy to recognize by the cat owner are discussed.

The use of homeopathic remedies is possible with a few disorders of the hormonal glands. Treatment, however, should be by an experienced therapist.

Malfunctions of the Thyroid Gland

Thyroid deficiency (hypothyroidism) is rare in cats; overactivity of this gland (hyperthyroidism) is more common.

Symptoms of deficiency: Stunted growth, constipation, subnormal temperature, reduced heart rate.

Symptoms of overactivity: Overexcitability, restlessness, voracious appetite, weight loss, increase in heart rate and cardiac activity (see "Health Check," page 11), enlarged thyroid (predominantly in old cats).

▪ Homeopathy with Skin Disorders

For dosages, see page 60.

Suppurations, Abscesses
- Acute reddening, heat, pain: *Hepar sulfuris.*
- After the acute phase: *Myristica sebifera.*
- Chronic suppurations, fistulas, poorly healing wounds: *Silicea.*
- Hard swelling, watery, foul-smelling secretion: *Mercurius solubilis.*
- Viscous, creamy pus: *Pulsatilla.*

Hint: See also "Homeopathy with Wounds and Injuries," page 73.

Eczema
- Dry eczema: *Arsenicum album,* sulfur, *Causticum, Natrium muriaticum.*
- Weeping eczema: *Arsenicum album, Cantharis, Mercurius solubilis, Silicea, Rhus toxicodendron.*
- Chronic eczema: *Lycopodium, Arsenicum album, Acidum formicicum.*

Miscellaneous Disorders
- Shaggy coat: Sulfur.
- Matted hair: *Acidum fluoricum.*
- Very dry coat: *Calcium carbonicum,* sulfur.
- Oily coat: *Natrium muriaticum,* sulfur.
- Brittle nails: *Silicea.*
- Flea allergy: *Acidum formicicum*
- Insect bites: *Apis*
- Burns: *Causticum.*

Causes:
- Hypothyroidism can be inherited or evoked by inflammations, injuries, and tumorous growths.
- Hypothyroidism results in increased metabolism through overproduction of thyroid hormones. A tumor can also be the cause.

● **Treatment**

▶ The veterinarian will make the diagnosis.
- With hypothyroidism a blood test is performed to determine whether a hormone deficiency is present. If so, the missing hormone (thyroxine) has to be supplied in the form of tablets.
- With hyperthyroidism the enlarged thyroid gland can be palpated. Radioactive iodine or Methimazole (to inhibit hormone production) is used as therapy. If that fails, the thyroid gland is removed.

Follow-up care: A cat with hypothyroidism needs to take hormone replacement tablets the rest of its life. They are added to its food each day. With hyperthyroidism the cat takes medications as directed by the veterinarian.

Adrenal Hyperfunction

Symptoms: Excessive thirst and increased urination, increased appetite, muscular atrophy, potbelly, dull coat, loss of hair over the trunk.

Causes: The tiny adrenal glands are located near the kidneys. The medulla of the adrenal (suprarenal) gland is distinct from the adrenal cortex. Important hormones, including adrenaline, are produced in the medulla. Its outer area (cortex) produces hormones (corticosteroids) that perform important functions in the metabolic process.

Hyperfuncton can be caused by a tumor of the adrenal cortex or by overproduction of ACTH, a hormone that is made in the pituitary gland (hypophysis) and acts on the adrenal glands.

This rare disease frequently goes hand in hand with diabetes.

● **Treatment**

▶ Exact diagnosis requires costly lab tests. Today smaller tumors can be treated surgically by veterinarians with promising results.

Adrenal Hypofunction

Symptoms: Apathy, dehydration, refusal to eat, frequent vomiting.

Causes: Diminished function because of injuries from accidents, infections, tumors, or shrinkage (atrophy) of the adrenal cortex. Hypofunction can also occur after prolonged treatment with cortisone or sex hormones (progesterone, see "Glossary," page 113).

Effects: Acute circulatory problems that can result in shock and sudden death.

- **Treatment**

▶ For exact diagnosis the veterinarian will employ special hormone-detection procedures. The dehydration is offset by infusions, and missing hormones are supplied in tablet form or by injection.

Follow-up care: Add tablets to the cat's food daily, as directed by veterinarian. Therapy is usually life-long. It is important for the cat to drink large amounts of water, so you need to add a pinch of table salt to its food (0.1 gram of table salt per 2.2 pounds [1 kg] of the cat's body weight).

Diabetes

Cats, too, can suffer from diabetes (*diabetes mellitus*), although it is far less common in cats than in humans.

Symptoms: Excessive thirst and frequent urination, increasing appetite, weight loss. These symptoms, however, may also be signs of other diseases.

Causes: Insulin, a hormone produced in the pancreas, is absent or can no longer be secreted in adequate amounts.

Effects: The blood sugar level soars as a result of insulin deficiency, and sugar is eliminated through the kidneys. The urine contains sugar. If the disease is not treated, serious consecutive damage is done to the liver and other organs, ultimately resulting in death.

- **Treatment**

▶ Possible only by the veterinarian. To make exact diagnosis possible the blood sugar level is determined on the basis of blood and urine samples.

In most cases a daily insulin injection is necessary for the remainder of the cat's life. The exact dose for an individual cat has to be determined by extensive testing.

A special diet is not essential, but you should divide your pet's daily ration into two servings.

Follow-up care: Life-long insulin injections on a daily basis, as directed by the veterinarian (see "Insulin Injections," page 52).

Deficiency of Sex Hormones

Disturbances in the sensitive hormonal-control systems always result in serious disease processes in cats. An exception is deficiency of sex hormones. In female and male cats the production of sex hormones comes practically to a standstill when the animals are altered. With respect to the well-being and life expectancy of the individual cat, altering even proves quite advantageous (see "Altering or Sterilization," page 24).

Among females used for breeding a deficiency of sex hormones may occasionally result in an undesirable absence of estrus, or heat. That can be remedied through hormone therapy.

In cats that live outdoors a break in the estrus cycle normally occurs during the inhospitable winter season.

Disorders of the Urinary Tract and Reproductive Organs

Urine is produced by the kidneys. It contains many waste products that the kidneys have filtered out of the blood. Through the ureters the urine collects in the bladder and is excreted via the urethra. The kidneys regulate the electrolyte and water balance and control important properties of the blood. In addition some hormones are produced in the kidneys.

Acute Kidney Failure

Symptoms: Decreased excretion of urine, increased thirst, refusal to eat, apathy, gastrointestinal upsets, vomiting. The symptoms are extremely diverse.

Causes:

- Shock, perhaps after an accident involving significant loss of blood.
- Blockage of the urinary passages by urethral and bladder stones.
- Retention of urine caused by urethral injuries and bladder rupture.
- Kidney infection.
- Poisoning by heavy metals (mercury, lead, cadmium, thallium, arsenic), antifreeze (glycol), or medications.

Effects: Acute kidney failure can be fatal.

● Treatment

▶ Go immediately to the veterinarian. In this emergency situation, the cat will be treated first with infusions and diuretics in order to get the kidneys working again. Then the exact cause has to be discovered.

Follow-up care: Complete healing of the underlying illness—for example, curing an infection with antibiotic therapy over the course of several weeks. In many cases a special diet for kidney problems (see page 22) is useful.

■ Homeopathy

See page 82.

Chronic Kidney Damage

Symptoms: Increased thirst and urination (pale, watery urine), breath that smells of urine, vomiting.

Causes: Many lesions of the kidney tissue—caused by infections, for example—precede chronic renal insufficiency. Elderly cats are especially affected.

Effects: Atrophy of the kidney leads to uremia (see "Glossary," page 113). Severe uremia results in death.

● Treatment

▶ Possible only by the veterinarian, who will examine the cat by palpating the kidneys. Urine and blood tests provide reliable information on the state of the disease. Treatment begins with infusions of electrolyte solutions (water, salts, glucose). A diet that contains reduced amounts of protein and phosphorus (see page 22) is required. All the procedures listed above merely slow down the disease process. When the cat begins to suffer, it should be put to sleep (see page 45).

Follow-up care: For the remainder of the cat's life a specially formulated diet for kidney problems. The cat needs to drink copious amounts of water. Add a pinch of table salt to your pet's food.

■ Homeopathy

See page 82.

Urinary Calculus (Feline Urological Syndrome, FUS)

Symptoms: Urination frequently accompanied by pain; urine sometimes mixed with crystals and blood; swelling and blue coloration of the tip of the penis, which the cat licks.

Causes: Formation of fine, sandy gravel or larger stones (concretions) in the urine.

These insoluble formations can give rise to inflammation in the urethra and also, by blocking the urethra, cause retention of urine. Infectious causes and hereditary predispositions are also possible.

According to the National Research Council (NRC), "inattention" to the effects of diet composition on the acid–base balance of the body "may be a major factor" in causing FUS. The "ingestion of abnormally large quantities of base-forming elements" by the cat—"an animal that has been ... adapted to produce acid urine" with a pH of 6.0 to 7.0—may be responsible for driving a cat's pH above the 7.1 level, where crystallization begins to occur spontaneously. The NRC cautions against pinning the blame for FUS on any particular mineral—magnesium, for example. (FUS affects males predominantly, because of their relatively long, narrow urethra.)

Effects: Urinary retention can, if the urethra is completely obstructed, progress through acute kidney failure (see page 80) and uremia to death.

● Treatment

▶ Possible only by the veterinarian. He or she first will palpate the bladder and examine the urinary aperture. If the diagnosis is confirmed, a urinary catheter is carefully pushed through the urethra into the bladder of the anesthetized cat.

Smaller urinary calculus can be removed in most cases by irrigation with an acid solution. Afterward the cat receives antibiotics and antispasmodics.

If the urethra is completely blocked and the bladder is in danger of rupturing, it is necessary to operate at once.

Even after successful treatment, it is possible for new stones to form.

Follow-up care: A life-long special diet for prevention of urinary calculus is usually required (commercial diet foods are available from veterinarians).

Make sure your pet's intake of liquids is adequate. Add a pinch of table salt to the cat's food.

Prevention: Always provide ample drinking water. Limit the food ration to one or two servings a day. Don't overfeed your cat.

■ Homeopathy

See page 82.

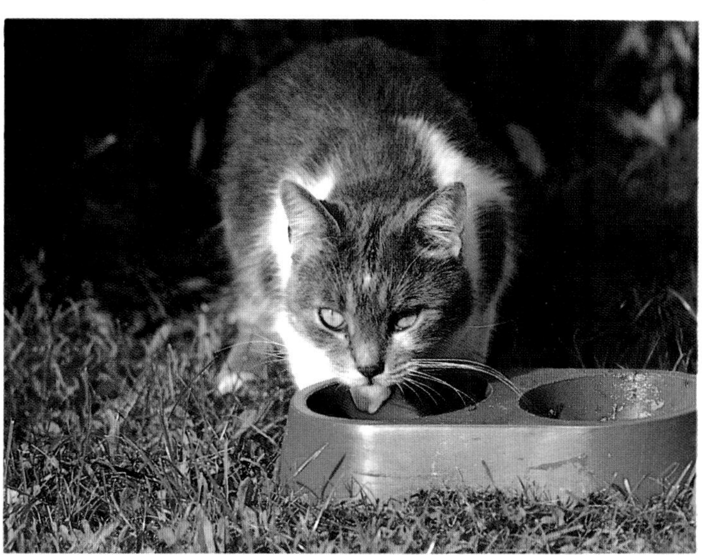

When its urinary system is diseased, a cat needs to drink copious amounts of water.

Bacterial Infection of the Urethra and Bladder

Symptoms: Decreased appetite, increased water intake, increased urination, blood in urine, cat seems apathetic and feels pain when abdomen is touched.

Causes: The infection, caused by bacteria, usually begins in the urethra and ascends to the bladder.

● Treatment

▶ Go to the veterinarian at once. He or she will make the diagnosis on the basis of a urine test or possibly after microbiological cultivation of the pathogens in question. Antibiotics help control urethritis and cystitis.

Follow-up care: Antibiotics for about three weeks (longer if the kidney is also affected). Add a pinch of table salt to the cat's food so that your pet will drink plenty of water.

■ Homeopathy

See above right.

Female Reproductive Disorders

The cat's paired ovaries are located in the abdominal cavity. In addition to providing sexual cells, they regulate reproduction through the production of sex hormones.

Homeopathy with Kidney and Bladder Disorders

For dosages, see page 60.

- No urine produced despite urge to urinate, urine produced only in drops, in some cases bloody: *Sabal serrulatum.*
- To promote kidney function: *Berberis, Solidago.*
- Urge to urinate, pain, involuntary urination: *Cantharis.*
- Urination with interrupted stream, dribbling: *Causticum.*
- Chronic disorders: *Arsenicum album.*

Hint: Always see the veterinarian immediately for any kidney or bladder problems.

Uterine Infection

Symptoms: In some cases mucopurulent discharge that soils the rear thighs; cat frequently licks these areas clean. Apathetic behavior, lack of appetite, fever, increased intake of water, vomiting, dehydration, dull coat; gradual distention of the abdomen.

Causes: An infection of the uterus (pyometra) can arise without causative pathogens (bacteria) being discovered. Frequently, however, bacterial pathogens can be found in the purulent discharge at the onset of the disease or during its course.

Uterine infection apparently is fostered by hormone treatments that suppress heat.

Effects: Life-threatening changes in the blood and damage to organs; the pus can penetrate into the abdominal cavity, causing infertility or peritonitis and possibly death.

● Treatment

▶ With all disorders of the ovaries and uterus the safest method of treatment is surgical removal of these organs. In exceptional cases, in young cats deemed especially valuable from a breeding standpoint, for example, pyometra in the early stage can be treated with antibiotics and special tissue hormones (prostaglandin preparations).

Follow-up care: Give antibiotics and tissue hormones (prostaglandins, see "Glossary," page 113) until healing is complete.

Prevention: Give as few hormone treatments as possible to breeding queens. Have your pet spayed if it is not used for breeding.

■ Homeopathy

See page 78.

Male Reproductive Disorders

Like other organs, the testicles also are subject to infections, tumors, and degeneration. With the exception of a small number of purebred studs, almost all well-cared-for males are castrated while young (see page 24). For that reason only the presence of testicles in the wrong place presents a significant problem.

Poorly Developed Testicles

Symptoms: The testicles are smaller than those of other male cats comparable in age.

Causes: Hereditary predisposition. As a rule the very rare tortoiseshell, or three-colored, males, are affected by defective development of the testicles (Chromosome constitution, see "Glossary," page 113). Very poorly developed testicles can be the result of a feline panleukopenia (FPL) infection before or shortly after birth (see page 107).

Effects: Diminished fertility.

Undescended Testicles

In the course of their development the testicles move from their original site in the abdominal cavity through the inguinal canal into the scrotum, which is located just under the anal opening.

Symptoms: If one or both testicles are retained in the abdominal cavity or in the inguinal canal, we say that the testicles have failed to descend. Only one testicle—or none at all—can be felt in the scrotum.

Causes: Hereditary predisposition. If both testicles are in the abdominal cavity (cryptorchidism), the cat is sterile but displays normal or even exaggerated sexual behavior. If only one testicle is in its normal place in the scrotum (monorchidism), neither the cat's sexual behavior nor its procreative capacity is impaired. In rare instances only one testicle is present in the first place.

Effects: Abdominal testicles allegedly promote tumor formation.

● **Treatment**

▶ The veterinarian will recommend castration (see page 24).

Prevention: Do not use male cats with monorchidism for breeding purposes.

Penile Adhesions

Symptoms: Decreased urination, which can be accompanied by symptoms similar to those of urinary tract infections (see page 81).

Causes: Castrating a male before the onset of puberty may promote adhesions between the penis and the prepuce. For this reason males should be castrated at roughly seven months of age.

Effects: Penile adhesions can lead to chronic inflammations.

● **Treatment**

▶ Go to the veterinarian.

• Adhesions can be surgically treated by the veterinarian.

• Inflammations (see "Bacterial Infection of the Urethra and Bladder," page 82).

■ **Homeopathy**

See page 78.

Infertility and Inability to Mate

The inability of a male cat to mate and/or to procreate is of importance only to breeders of purebred cats. Disorders of mating behavior can result from various diseases or mental problems (for example, if the male is placed in an unfamiliar environment to mate with a female).

Sterility too can be caused by disease, but it may be hereditary as well. If the cat is unable to mate, behavioral therapy is possible.

Sterile males should be castrated (see "Altering or Sterilization," page 24).

5 Disorders of the Digestive System

Diseases that affect the gastrointestinal tract, the liver, and the pancreas generally present one or more of the following symptoms: diarrhea, constipation, vomiting, and lack of appetite. These problems tell us nothing for the moment about the degree of severity of the disorder. Often they can be remedied easily or they disappear without treatment. Sometimes, however, they signal the onset of a serious, life-threatening, or even incurable disease.

Problems Caused by Foreign Bodies

Symptoms: Depending on the location of the foreign body, spasmodic jaw movements, choking, and wiping with the forepaws, heavy drooling, vomiting; if the cat is in pain, it quits eating.

Causes:

- A piece of bone has become wedged between the teeth in the oral cavity.
- Needles can get stuck in the cat's tongue or the back of its throat. Usually they were pulled in when the cat chewed on the attached thread.
- Other foreign bodies (buttons, plastic parts) are swallowed into the stomach, but their size prevents them from traveling any farther into the intestine.
- Some foreign bodies (marbles, tinsel) can pass through the pylorus but then get stuck and cause a life-threatening intestinal blockage.
- Drooling, especially if accompanied by abnormal behavior, might be a sign of rabies.

● **Treatment**

▶ If there are grounds for suspicion, go the veterinarian immediately. Removal of foreign bodies in the oral cavity usually is possible only under anesthesia. With objects that have been swallowed, a radiograph can provide information. In many cases the veterinarian has to operate.

Prevention: Do not leave anything lying around that could be dangerous for the cat.

Vomiting

Symptoms: Occasional vomiting is frequently accompanied by noises resembling coughing and by apparent convulsions.

Causes: Cats by nature are very prone to vomiting. Many cats ingest grass or plant parts for that very purpose. Vomiting up the contents of its stomach is a cat's way of getting rid of unwholesome or indigestible food as quickly as possible.

● **Treatment**

Occasional vomiting is completely normal in cats.

▶ If vomiting occurs more frequently—for example, every

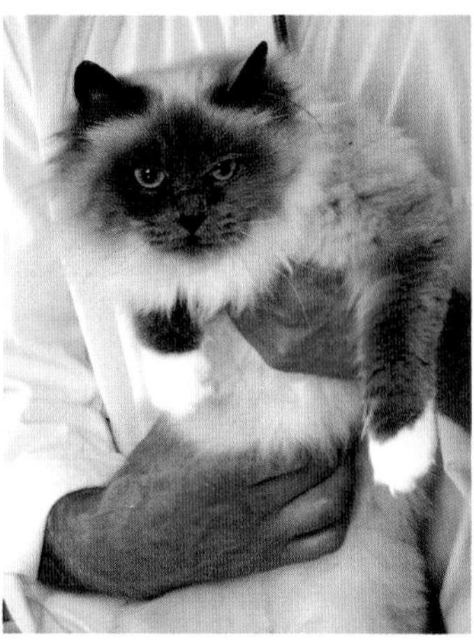

The veterinarian is palpating this cat's abdomen.

time the cat has eaten—a serious disorder is present; the cat has to be examined by the veterinarian.

■ **Homeopathy**
See page 86.

Diarrhea

Symptoms: Watery feces, frequently an unimpaired general state of health for the time being, apathy, dehydration if diarrhea persists, dull coat.

Causes: The diarrhea may perform a protective function if it is a way of quickly expelling harmful intestinal contents. In many cases, however, it is the result of a disease process. Possible causes are consumption of indigestible food, acute or chronic inflammations, parasite infestation, or infectious diseases (for example, feline panleukopenia, discussed on page 107).

Effects: Continued diarrhea always results in dehydration of the cat's body. Dehydration is present if you can make a fold in the cat's coat between two fingers and it does not smooth out again as soon as you let it go. The loss of water, electrolytes, and protein can lead to death.

● **Treatment**

If the cat's overall health and behavior are normal, there is no cause to worry for the time being.

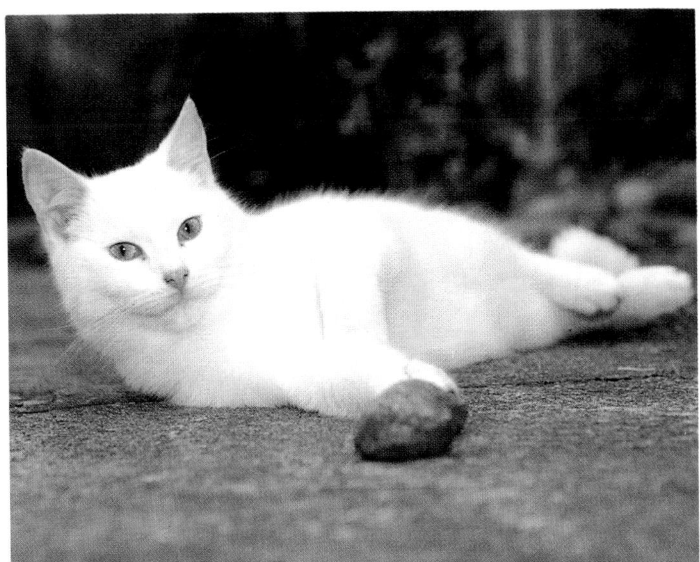

If the cat is feeling fine, there is no immediate cause for concern if diarrhea occurs.

In many cases the cat will be cured if you immediately stop feeding it and deny it food for one to two days. It is important that the cat have clean, fresh drinking water available at all times. After the period of withholding food place the cat on a special diet. In young cats especially any disturbance of bowel function tends to be expressed in the form of diarrhea.

Diet recipe: Two parts cottage cheese and one part boiled rice or mashed potatoes prepared without milk. Serve only very small portions (one heaping tablespoonful) four times a day, freshly prepared each time. After a few days the cottage cheese can be replaced with boiled chicken or lamb. Gradually make the switch back to the cat's usual food.

Important: Never try to control your pet's diarrhea by denying it drinking water. The body loses a great deal of fluid through diarrhea and vomiting. If the water loss is not replaced, the cat can die. If it obviously is drinking too little, add a pinch of salt to the special diet food.

▶ If, despite all your efforts, the diarrhea recurs, you need to consult the veterinarian at once so that he or she can determine and treat the causes.

If dehydration is occurring, the cat will be given an infusion immediately.

■ **Homeopathy**
See below.

Inflammation of the Stomach Lining (Gastritis)

Symptoms: Listlessness, refusal to eat, vomiting.

Causes: Gastritis can be caused by impurities and irritants (indigestible medications, foreign bodies in the stomach, poisoning, spoiled food) or various infectious diseases. Gastritis where kidney failure is present is a special form.

Usually gastritis is linked with inflammation in the intestines (enteritis).

Effects: Electrolyte (see "Glossary," page 113) and fluid loss can create a life-threatening situation.

● **Treatment**

▶ Only the veterinarian can determine the exact cause.

- For acute gastritis, see "Follow-up care," below.
- Chronic gastritis requires a special test.

Follow-up care: If the veterinarian's diagnosis is acute gastritis, let the cat fast for one to two days, then feed it a bland diet of boiled rice with a 5 percent glucose solution (available from the veterinarian).

Prevention: Never give your pet food that is too hot or too cold.

■ **Homeopathy**
See below.

Constipation

Symptoms: Failure to pass stool, straining with no success, restlessness, apathy, gradual increase in abdominal girth.

■ Homeopathy with Disorders of the Digestive Organs

For dosages, see page 60.

- Results of wrong food, too much food, or spoiled food: *Nux vomica.*
- Constipation, urge to go but without success: *Nux vomica.*
- Sluggish bowels: *Nux vomica* together with *Carbo vegetabilis.*
- Acid diarrhea, milk not tolerated: *Calcium carbonicum.*
- Sensitive stomach, vomiting up of undigested food: *Ipecacuanha.*
- Severe, watery diarrhea: *Podophyllum.*
- Vomiting after eating or drinking: Phosphorus.
- Alternating diarrhea and constipation: Sulfur.

Causes: Infections, paralysis of the bowels, hair balls or bezoars (see "Glossary," page 113), worms, and tumors. Food that is very low in roughage promotes the syndrome (see "Proper Nutrition," page 16).

Sometimes feces that adhere near the anus (especially in neglected longhaired cats and in kittens) blocks the passage of stool.

Effects: Intestinal obstruction (see page 87).

● **Treatment**

If feces are clinging to the anal area, see "How-to: Preventive Care," page 14.

▶ The veterinarian has to determine the exact causes of the constipation. He or she can detect the fecal concretions by palpation. To soften them and induce the passage of stool, the cat is given mineral oil and enemas. Pure water cannot be used to give a cat an enema because it can cause breaking down of the blood (hemolysis).

If the treatment is not successful, the abdomen has to be opened in order to provide relief through direct massage of the bowels and to remove hair balls, worm clusters, or tumors. To prevent infection, the cat is given several injections of antibiotics.

Follow-up care: In some cases give enemas as directed by the veterinarian until the cat has a bowel movement. After surgery, check-ups by the veterinarian.

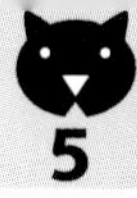

Prevention: Roughage in the cat's food (add some bran).

- **Homeopathy**
  See page 86.

Inflammation of the Bowel

Symptoms: Listlessness, refusal to eat, vomiting, diarrhea, dehydration.

Causes: Enteritis (inflammation of the small intestine) resulting from parasite infestation (see "Disorders Caused by Parasites," page 96) is especially common in young cats.

Nutrition-related inflammations of the bowels occur primarily in cats that live outdoors. Allergies and, in some cases, incurable viral infections can also be caused (see "Infectious Diseases," page 104).

Effects: Chronic inflammation of the bowel (right).

- **Treatment**

Have cat fast for at least one day, then use a special diet (see "Diarrhea," page 85).

▶ If there is no improvement and the cat vomits frequently, continues to have diarrhea despite the special diet, and is apathetic, it has to be taken to the veterinarian at once.

To compensate for the fluid loss the cat will first be given an infusion. The vet will prescribe antispasmodic medications (spasmolytics) and antiemetics (see "Glossary," page 113).

- With severe infections treatment with antibiotics.
- With allergic processes use of corticosteroids (see "Glossary," page 113).

Prevention: Don't give your pet food that is cold or spoiled. Make sure the cat remains free of parasites.

- **Homeopathy**
  See page 86.

Chronic Inflammation of the Bowel

Symptoms: Variable stool consistency and color (usually liquid or thin and runny with mucus or blood) over a prolonged period, varying appetite, weight loss, dehydration, apathy. In some cases, however, diarrhea is the only sign of ill health.

Causes: Consequences of an acute inflammation of the bowel. Severe, incurable forms often are caused by specific viral infections. Liver and pancreatic diseases also result in chronic disorders.

- **Treatment**

Once the cause has been found, the therapy will be based on it. General dietary measures as with the acute form of the disease.

If dehydration and weight loss are present, appropriate adjunct therapy. If a disorder turns out to be incurable, the cat should be put to sleep.

- **Homeopathy**
  See page 86.

Paralysis of the Bowel

Symptoms: Decreased defecation, retention of stool in bowel, lack of appetite, vomiting, drying out of the body.

Causes: Neural and vascular damage, incurable diseases (for example, feline leukemia virus disease, discussed on page 106).

Effects: Untreated paralysis of the bowel results in death.

- **Treatment**

▶ The veterinarian will make the diagnosis. To make up for the lost fluid, the cat will be given infusions and medications to stimulate the bowels.

Intestinal Obstruction (Blocked Bowel)

Symptoms: General ill health, loss of appetite, failure to pass stool, vomiting.

Causes: An intestinal obstruction can come about as a result of all the disease processes previously described in this chapter.

Effects: Untreated intestinal obstruction results in death.

● **Treatment**

▶ The veterinarian will make the diagnosis. Radiographs (after the cat has been given a barium meal) can be helpful for that purpose. An intestinal obstruction has to be treated surgically.

Follow-up care: The veterinarian will check on the healing of the incision.

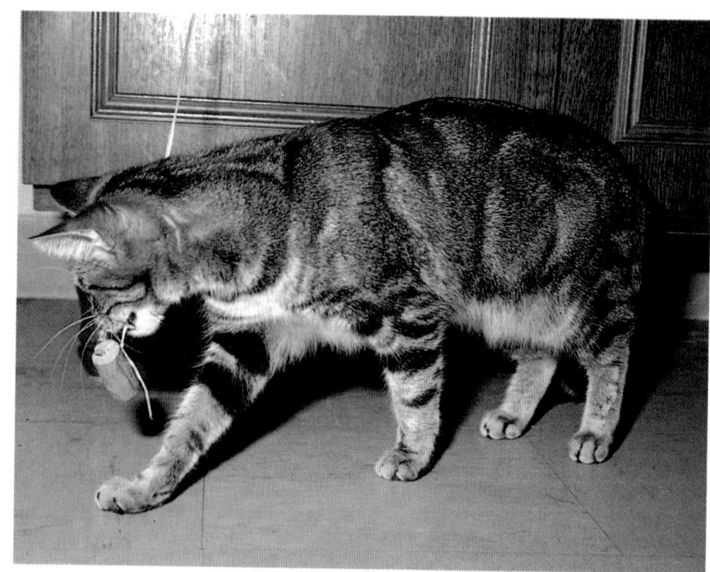

It is fine for the cat to play with the cork under supervision. But if a cat swallows an indigestible object, intestinal obstruction can result.

Liver Disease

The liver is irreplaceable in the metabolic process. It functions as a detoxification and storage organ, and converts vitamins and hormones. For these reasons liver diseases and damage manifest themselves in many different ways.

Symptoms: The cat seems exhausted and listless, refuses to eat, has a dull coat; drooling, vomiting, diarrhea.

Key symptoms: Jaundice or icterus (see "Glossary," page 113), enlarged liver, light-colored, pale-yellowish feces, dark-brown urine.

Causes:

• Inflammations (infectious and noninfectious). Acute liver inflammations can be caused by infectious agents (viruses, bacteria, fungi, parasites) or by poisons.

• A fatty liver results primarily from overweight.

• Rarely, tumors of the liver, which usually are malignant. These are predominantly metastases (see "Glossary," page 113) of tumors (for example, FeLV tumors).

Liver disease may be acute or chronic. Chronic liver damage can be caused by infections, congestion due to cardiac insufficiency (see page 94), gradual poisoning of the blood, hormonal disorders, or tumors.

Effects: The final stage of many liver diseases is cirrhosis (degeneration of the liver tissue).

● **Treatment**

▶ Possible only by the veterinarian. The exact diagnosis is based on blood tests (hepatic values, increase of specific enzymes) or a biopsy.

As an emergency measure intravenous feeding. Then, treatment of the primary disease—with bacterial infections, for example, antibiotic therapy for three weeks.

With acute and chronic diseases as soon as the cat can eat on its own again, give it a highly nutritious diet, free of harmful substances and rich in protein. Suitable foods include cottage cheese and boiled rice, enriched with a vitamin and mineral supplement. Commercial diet foods are also available from veterinarians (see "Special Diets," page 22).

Follow-up care: Antibiotics for up to three weeks, strict diet formulated for liver problems, regular checking of hepatic values by the veterinarian.

■ **Homeopathy**
Carduus marianus, Chelidonium, Lycopodium, sulfur, phosphorus, Flor de Pieda, *Nux vomica.*

Pancreatic Disease

Besides hormone production the most important task of the pancreas is the production, storage, and secretion of digestive enzymes (see "Glossary," page 113).

Symptoms: Lack of appetite, weakness, increased intake of water, frequent urination, diarrhea, constipation, and vomiting.

Causes: Infections that originate in the intestines and injury (after a serious accident). Inflammations of the pancreas (pancreatitis) are not common in cats. There is a chronic form of pancreatitis that starts in the structural tissue and often presents no noticeable symptoms for a long while. In the course of an acute inflammation the digestive enzymes are activated prematurely, and the organ begins to digest itself.

● **Treatment**
▶ Possible only by the veterinarian, who will make an exact diagnosis based on blood tests. If the pancreas is failing, fat can be detected in the stool. In an acute case the cat can no longer ingest food; it has to be fed intravenously until the inflammation subsides.

With chronic inflammation all one can do is combat the symptoms. A special low-fat diet (available from the veterinarian) supports the treatment.

Anal Sac Infection

This condition is rare in cats.

Symptoms: Reddened and swollen anal sacs, which the cat frequently licks and nibbles.

Causes and effects: The anal sacs can become impacted by glandular hypersecretion (secretion, see "Glossary," page 113). That causes them to become inflamed and to swell on one or both sides of the anus.

The cat's licking and nibbling often result in the development of eczema or pus-producing fistulas.

● **Treatment**
▶ Possible only by the veterinarian. Often, expressing and irrigating the anal sacs with a 2 percent hydrogen peroxide solution is possible only if the cat is under anesthesia. Afterward, several weeks of treatment with antibiotics.

Follow-up care: Antibiotics as directed by the veterinarian.

■ **Homeopathy**
See page 78.

Rectal and Anal Prolapse

Symptoms: The mucous membrane of the rectum bulges out of the anus in the form of a gelatinous, bluish red protuberance.

Causes: Caused by a weakness of the anal sphincter in the course of inflammatory processes.

● **Treatment**
▶ Go to the veterinarian immediately. In mild cases the rectal mucous membrane can be pushed back into the anus. In some cases an operation is required.

Follow-up care: Several weekly follow-up examinations by the veterinarian. In the first few days make sure that the cat's stool is soft (give your pet raw liver or some milk). The veterinarian can also provide you with a high-energy paste that you can feed the cat temporarily.

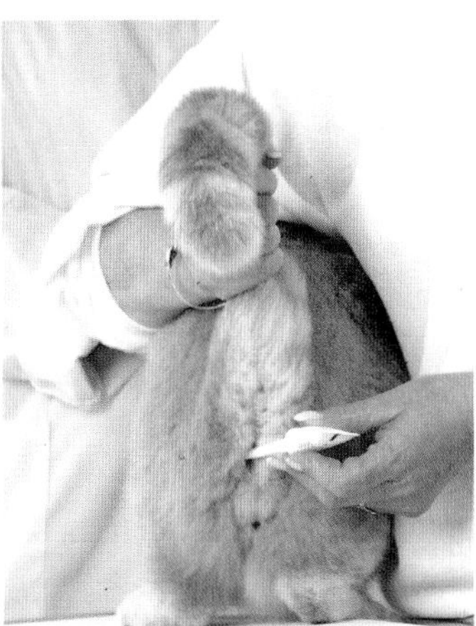

A cat with constipation is given enemas to induce the passage of stool.

6 Disorders of the Respiratory and Circulatory Systems

During inhalation, air travels through the cat's oral and nasal cavities, larynx, trachea, and bronchial tubes into its lungs. Enriched there with oxygen, the blood then flows to the heart and is pumped through the aorta and the arteries into the body. The depleted, oxygen-poor blood flows through the veins back to the heart and from there to the lungs again, where it once more is enriched with oxygen. Nutrients, water, and hormones are transported via the circulatory system.

Diseases in the Nose Area

Symptoms: Frequent sneezing, nasal discharge.

Causes: In cats the nose and throat area is often subject to infectious inflammatory processes, which in the broadest sense can be attributed to the "feline respiratory disease complex" and other infections (see "Feline Respiratory Disease," page 107).

- Irritations due to foreign bodies or allergies are rare.
- In animals with weakened immune systems a dangerous fungal infection also can occur on occasion (cryptococcosis).
- In isolated cases also caused by benign neoplasms or, even more rarely, by malignant tumors in the nose area.
- Occasionally an abscessed tooth root can cause these symptoms.

● Treatment

▶ Every cat with symptoms of respiratory disease should be taken to the veterinarian. In unclear cases microbiological testing of the nasal discharge can provide additional information.

Therapy for:

- infectious diseases (see page 104)
- allergies (see page 77)
- fungal infestation (see page 111)
- tumors (see "Nosebleed," right).

■ Homeopathy

See pages 78 and 91.

Nosebleed

Causes: As a consequence of accidents (a car accident, a fall from a great height), severe infections, or coagulatory disorders (for example, coumarin poisoning); sometimes attributable to a foreign body or a tumor in the nose.

● Treatment

▶ The veterinarian has to identify the cause.

- With bleeding caused by an accident the animal is kept quiet with medications. Compresses made with cold water or ice cubes can halt the bleeding.
- Infections (see "Infectious Diseases," page 104).
- With coumarin poisoning administer Vitamin K.

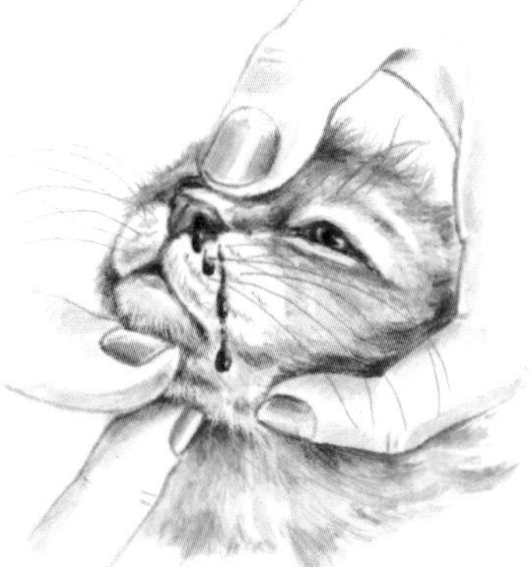

Nosebleed after injury.

• Foreign bodies and tumors have to be removed surgically.

Laryngitis

Symptoms: Coughing, hoarseness.

Causes: Viral infection (see "Feline Respiratory Disease," page 107), irritants, or foreign body. Incessant meowing (for example, during prolonged heat, discussed on page 36) can also lead to laryngitis.

● **Treatment**

▶ The veterinarian will determine the presence of laryngitis by examining the area at the back of the throat. He or she will detect reddening, swelling, or coatings. Depending on the severity of the case, expectorants, cortisone (see "Glossary" page 113), or antibiotics will be used for treatment.

Follow-up care: Until the cat recovers it has to be kept in a quiet room (see illustration, page 51).

Give medications as directed by veterinarian.

■ **Homeopathy**

See below.

Inflammation of the Pleura (Pleurisy)

Symptoms: Difficulty in breathing, fever, apathy.

Causes: If an inflammatory process develops on the fine membranes between which gliding movement of the respiratory organ is possible, we use the term pleurisy. The cause may include bacterial infections, injuries to the chest wall, and tears in the throat caused by foreign bodies.

Effects: Permanent damage with difficulty in breathing, death. A special, incurable form can develop as a result of an FIP infection (see page 104).

● **Treatment**

▶ The veterinarian has to identify the cause. Radiographs (see "Glossary," page 113), blood tests, and fine-needle aspiration of the thoracic cavity are helpful tools. If the condition is bacterial in origin, antibiotics are used in addition to the supporting therapy (infusions, immobilization). The disease is serious, and the prospects of recovery are not good.

■ **Homeopathy**

See pages 63 and left.

■ Homeopathy with Respiratory Disorders

For dosages, see page 60.

Nose

• Stuffy nose, almost no discharge: *Hepar sulfuris.*

• Tearing eyes, sneezing, watery cold: *Cepa.*

• Nasal discharge thick, creamy: *Pulsatilla.*

• Nasal discharge light yellow, viscous: *Kalium bichromaticum.*

• Nasal discharge yellowish green: *Lycopodium.*

• Chronic problems: *Silicea.*

Hint: See also the homeopathic recommendations on page 78.

Cough

• Spasmodic coughing: *Belladonna, Drosea, Cuprum sulfuricum, Ipecacuanha.*

• Coughing that gets worse in warm rooms: *Pulsatilla, Natrium muriaticum.*

• Coughing, especially after excitement: *Chamomilla.*

• Coughing to the point of vomiting: *Ipecacuanha, Cuprum sulfuricum, Drosera, Belladonna.*

Inflammation of the Trachea and Bronchial Tubes

Symptoms: Deep, often whistling cough. The cat can do virtually nothing, tires quickly, and, as the disease progresses, suffers from difficulty in breathing, especially in exhalation.

Causes: Acute or chronic inflammation of the trachea and bronchial tubes is usually accompanied by inflammation of the larynx and throat area.

Often a bacterial infection is the cause. Mucus increasingly collects in the bronchial tubes, and in connection with an inflammation of the mucosa it can lead to obstruction of individual bronchial tubes. The characteristic cough is primarily a way of freeing the respiratory passages by getting the mucus out.

Effects: The acute disease can turn into chronic tracheobronchitis (tracheal and bronchial inflammation).

● **Treatment**

▶ Possible only by the veterinarian. The bacterial infection is controlled with broad-spectrum antibiotics (effective against many kinds of bacteria). In addition, medications are available that expand the bronchial tubes and liquefy the viscous mucus. Cortisone is also used, especially with chronic cases.

Follow-up care: Until recovery, medications as directed by the veterinarian. Let the cat inhale a chamomile solution once a day to speed the healing process. For this treatment place the animal in a pet carrier and close the door. Prepare a chamomile solution with hot water, put it into a small bowl, and set it in front of the carrier. Use a towel to help fan the vapors of the chamomile solution into the carrier. The chamomile vapors will give the cat relief when its respiratory passages are inflamed.

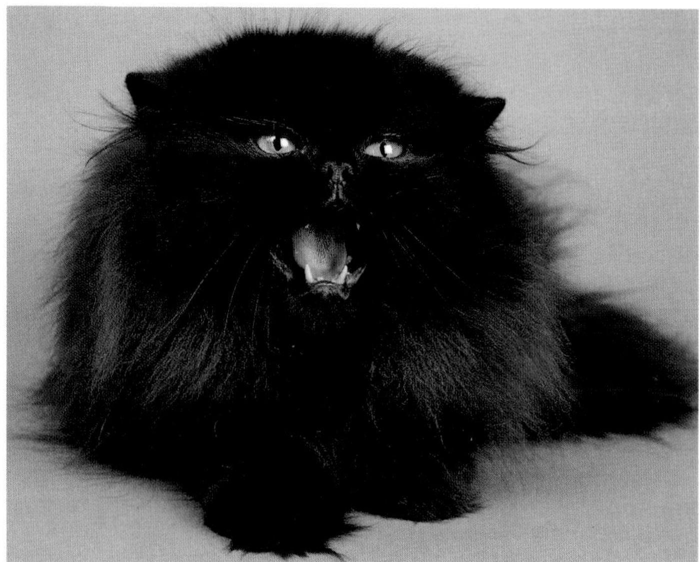

Persian cats can have difficulty breathing because of their noses, made short by selective breeding.

■ **Homeopathy**
See page 91.

Bronchial Asthma (Allergic Bronchitis)

Symptoms: Sudden onset of difficulty in breathing, strenuous coughing; occasionally the mucous membranes turn blue from lack of oxygen in the blood.

Causes: Allergic reaction to various substances (for example, pollen and household dust) can lead to a convulsive contraction of the bronchia.

● **Treatment**

▶ Possible only by the veterinarian. Cortisone is used for the treatment. With allergic reactions life-long therapy is often required.

■ **Homeopathy**
See page 91.

Air in the Pleural Cavity (Pneumothorax)

Symptoms: Pumping breathing, accelerated pulse, bluish coloring of tongue and mucous membranes.

Causes: Air can get into the space between the pleura and the pleura pulmonalis if a

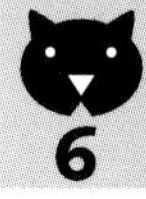

hole has formed in the lung and the pleura plumonalis or if the thoracic cage is open to the outside. The causes are small tears in the lung tissue, which often close on their own, or a penetration of the thoracic cage resulting from an accident.

● **Treatment**

▶ Go to the veterinarian at once. He or she will use radiographs to ascertain how much air has accumulated in the thorax. In mild cases nothing is done because within ten days the body will absorb the air that has made its way into the thorax.

If the thoracic cage has been pierced, the wound is closed to keep air out, and the air inside is extracted so that the lung can expand once more. Sometimes an operation is necessary. The cat is given antibiotics to prevent inflammation.

Follow-up care: Keep the cat in a quiet room on a warm bed (see page 51).

Ruptured Diaphragm

Symptoms: Difficulty in breathing with strenuous abdominal respiration, possibly vomiting.

Causes: Tears in the diaphragm usually result from car accidents. Depending on the site and size of the rupture, various organs in the abdominal cavity (portions of intestine, liver, stomach, spleen) can prolapse through this aperture into the chest cavity.

● **Treatment**

▶ Go to the veterinarian immediately. The nature and extent of the injuries can be determined from radiographs. Depending on the site of the individual case, surgery may be required.

During the operation artificial respiration is applied to the cat because the chest cavity has to be opened. To prevent inflammation: antibiotic therapy.

Follow-up care: Antibiotics for about one week.

Inflammation of the Lungs

Symptoms: High fever, apathy, refusal to eat.

Causes: The term *lung inflammation* (pneumonia) is used when the pulmonary functional tissue, the tiniest branches of the bronchial tree, or the intercalated supporting tissue are affected by the disease process. The causes include viruses, bacteria, fungi, and parasites. The bacterial diseases are of greatest significance for cats. Lung inflammation usually develops from bronchitis.

Effects: Permanent lung damage, death.

● **Treatment**

▶ The veterinarian will determine the extent, nature, and cause of the lung inflammation by auscultation (listening with a stethoscope), by testing secretions, and possibly by taking radiographs. Treatment with antibiotics. As an adjunct infusions are used to treat dehydration and to liquefy the bronchial secretion. For further treatment see "Inflammation of the Trachea and Bronchial Tubes," page 91.

Follow-up care: As for inflammation of the trachea and bronchial tubes (see page 91).

■ **Homeopathy**

See pages 63 and 91.

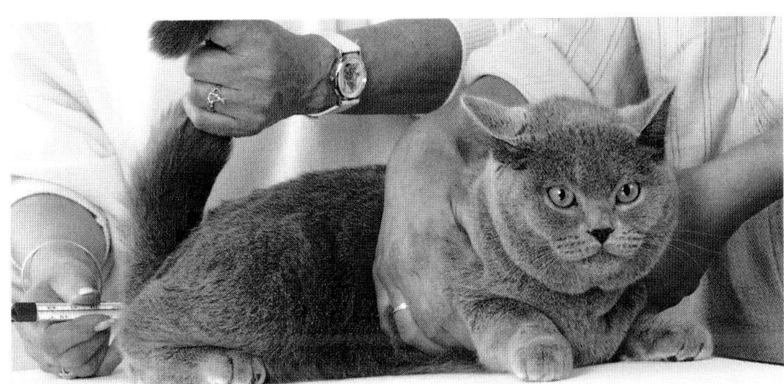

Taking a cat's temperature is really a job for two people (see page 50).

Pulmonary Edema

Symptoms: Shortness of breath, coughing, white foam that wells out of the nose, bluish colored mucous membranes, irregular, accelerated pulse.

Causes: Emergence of fluid into the air space of the lungs. The cause is usually a heart defect, but it can also be an allergy or a chemical irritation.

Effects: Death from suffocation.

● Treatment

▶ The veterinarian will treat the cat with sedative medications, cardiac and circulatory tonics, and diuretics (see "Glossary," page 113). If need be, respiration with oxygen.

Follow-up care: Medications as directed by the veterinarian.

Prevention: With cardiac insufficiency avoid excitement, exertion, excess weight, and heat.

■ Homeopathy

See above right.

Lung Tumors

Lung tumors, which usually do not originate in the lung itself, are metastases (see "Glossary," page 113). Once they reach a certain size (5 millimeters across), lung tumors can be detected in a radiograph. As a rule surgery is not performed. As long as the cat is feeling relatively well and is not yet having serious difficulty breathing, you can help it with restorative (anabolic) remedies (available from the veterinarian). If the cat is suffering, however, you should have the veterinarian put your pet to sleep (see page 45).

Heart and Circulatory Disorders

Symptoms: Apathetic behavior, decreased exercise tolerance, refusal to eat, great difficulty breathing when under strain, bluish or pallid coloration of mucous membranes.

Causes: Heart muscle (myocardial) damage and rhythm disorders or functional breakdowns of the valve flaps.

Often a cat is able to compensate for a gradually progressing cardiac insufficiency (inadequate performance of the heart) for a long while, unnoticed by anyone, because for the time being the heart is still performing well enough, provided the cat avoids physical stress. Overweight and old cats are most often affected.

Effects: Impairment of various organs and tissue—for example, congestion in the lung or liver, pulmonary edema (see left).

● Treatment

▶ Possible only by the veterinarian, who will diagnose heart defects by auscultation, taking the cat's pulse, and looking at radiographs and EKG results. In most cases no cure is possible, but the heart can be strengthened by medications. If the cardiac muscle is weak and the valve flaps are damaged, digitalis glycosides (see "Glossary," page 113) are used to boost myocardial efficiency. Diuretics (medications that increase urination) decrease congestion of tissues throughout the body, including the lungs and abdomen.

A low-sodium diet is easy on the heart (diet foods available from veterinarians).

Follow-up care: Medications have to be given for the remainder of the cat's life. Make sure your pet avoids physical overexertion. Always divide the special-diet food into small portions—about four servings per day.

Prevention: Nutritionally balanced diet (see page 16). Encourage indoor cats to get enough exercise.

■ Homeopathy

See above.

Homeopathy to Strengthen Circulation

For dosages, see page 60.

To support circulation during serious illnesses or after operations, to provide support in old cats: *Crataegus.*

Congenital Heart Defects

Heart defects can lead to premature death, or they can manifest themselves at first in the form of developmental disorders, stunted growth, and inactivity. Operations are possible and are within the budgets of many cat owners.

Thrombosis

Symptoms: In serious cases difficulty in breathing, shock, paralysis.

Causes: Blood clots (*thrombi*) in the blood vessels, often brought on by cardiomyopathy. If they are torn loose and carried in the bloodstream into the next capillary region, an embolism results from the obstruction of the narrow vessels.

Effects: Cerebral vascular stroke, renal infarction, leg paralysis, death.

● Treatment

No treatment is available for the cardiomyopathy that caused the thrombus, but in some cases thrombi can be removed surgically and in other cases the body is able to utilize alternate blood vessels to supply the region.

Blood

The blood is made up of blood plasma and blood cells. Most blood cells are anuclear red corpuscles, which transport oxygen with their hemoglobin. The white corpuscles are present in much smaller numbers. They serve to ward off pathogenic organisms. The blood is a means of transport for all vital substances.

Anemia

Anemia is the term applied to a deficiency of red blood cells and/or hemoglobin in the blood.

Symptoms: Pallid mucous membranes, decreased stress tolerance.

Causes: Heavy loss of blood after accidents; destruction of red blood cells because of infections, parasites, poisoning, and autoimmune-related diseases (see page 109); insufficient supply of red blood cells stemming from iron deficiency; severe liver and kidney damage or bone marrow impairment due to tumors, hormones, or medications; hereditary predisposition.

Effects: Anemia can be fatal.

● Treatment

Apply a pressure dressing (see page 54) as a first-aid measure to prevent heavy loss of blood after accidents, or tie off the affected limb.

▶ Then go immediately to the veterinarian.

- With heavy blood loss see right.
- Chronic anemia is analyzed on the basis of blood tests. The treatment depends on the underlying cause.

Follow-up care and prevention: Prevent iron deficiency by giving your cat a healthy diet (see page 16). If there is a hereditary predisposition, do not use the animal for breeding.

Blood Loss

Symptoms: Pallid mucous membranes, apathy, shock (loss of consciousness).

Effects: A normal cat (7.7 pounds [3.5 kg]) has about 8.5 fluid ounces (250 ml) of blood. A 10 percent blood loss (.85 fluid ounces [25 ml]) can be compensated for without difficulty. Clear signs of anemia (see left) do not appear until a loss of about 1.7 fluid ounces (50 ml) has occurred. With acute blood loss, 50 ml or more, because of an accident, symptoms of shock will appear.

● Treatment

▶ See "Anemia," left.

Severe blood loss is compensated for by blood transfusions from blood donors—other cats whose blood has been tested previously.

7 Disorders Caused by Parasites

Parasites are creatures that exist at the expense of their hosts and utilize the hosts' systems in order to live and reproduce. Ectoparasites (external parasites) are found on the body of the host; endoparasites (internal parasites), inside the host's body. Only the most common external and internal parasites of cats are discussed in this chapter.

Ear Mites

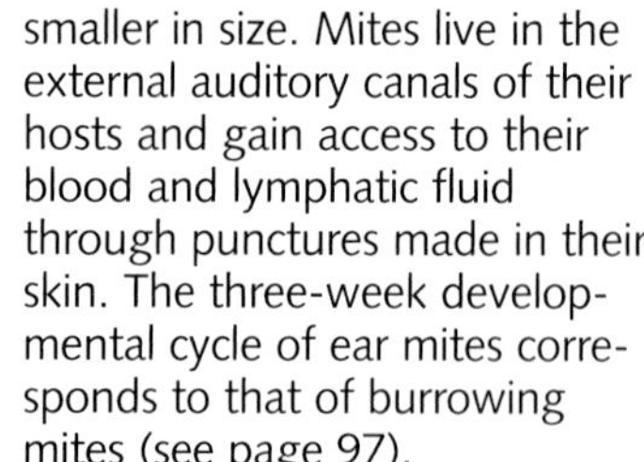

Female ear mites can reach a size of 0.5 millimeters, while males remain smaller in size. Mites live in the external auditory canals of their hosts and gain access to their blood and lymphatic fluid through punctures made in their skin. The three-week developmental cycle of ear mites corresponds to that of burrowing mites (see page 97).

Infestation: Usually through direct contact. Ear mites are not transmitted to humans.

Detection: Ear mites lay their eggs in the cat's ear canal. The mites' secretions, feces, and dead bodies form a crumbly, crusty substance there. The cat is tormented by severe itching, which causes it to shake its head and scratch at its ear constantly. The scratching, in turn, can cause pus-producing skin inflammations or even abscesses.

Effects: Inflammations develop in the ear canal, and in young cats their growth can be so severe that the ear canals are completely obstructed by plugs. The dirty substance in the auditory canal or the plug forms a breeding ground for fungi or bacteria, which can prolong the inflammatory process. In isolated cases, a severe inflammation can entail complications when the middle ear or even the inner ear becomes involved (see page 68).

● Treatment

▶ Using an otoscope (see "Glossary," page 113), the veterinarian can look at the ear canals and diagnose mite infestation. If there is any doubt, a sample is taken and examined under the microscope. The crusts in the ear are softened with an ear-cleaning solution, and the auditory canal is cleaned with a cotton-tipped applicator. The veterinarian will prescribe a miticidal and anti-inflammatory ointment.

There are many different products available, therefore the treatment regime may vary. In many cases a general anesthetic and an ear flush procedure at the veterinary hospital are the fastest, most effective, and painless way to treat the infection.

Follow-up care: Continue treatment with the medication as directed by your veterinarian.

If you own several cats, you have to treat all of them at the same time. Crusts that are hurled out when the cat shakes its head contain mites that will survive for weeks. They can cause a new infection, therefore your veterinarian may suggest a preparation to treat the environment as well.

Prevention: Inspect your pet's ears regularly.

■ Homeopathy

See page 78.

Burrowing Mites

Female burrowing mites can grow to a length of 0.3 millimeters, males, to 1.5 millimeters. The entire developmental cycle of burrowing mites takes place in the cat's skin. From the eggs deposited in the skin, a new generation of sexually mature animals develops in about three weeks, after going through one larval stage and two nymph stages.

Infestation: Through direct contact with another animal; weakened cats with impaired immune systems are especially susceptible.

Detection: Advanced mange can be recognized by the symptoms described below. In the initial stage exact diagnosis is made by the veterinarian by means of skin samples that are examined under the microscope to detect mites and mite eggs.

Symptoms and effects: Burrowing mites cause far-reaching skin destruction and severe inflammations by tunneling in the skin and by means of the waste products they eliminate.

At first, reddening, nodules, and pustules develop, eventually turning into gray, fissured crusts and bloody, pus-filled exudates (see "Glossary," page 113). We distinguish between head mange and overall mange, which can affect the entire body. Untreated animals become weaker and weaker and finally perish miserably.

Risk to humans: In rare cases burrowing mites can also be transmitted to humans, producing symptoms of mange.

- **Treatment**

Bathe and massage mildly affected cats with miticides (available in pet stores and from veterinarians). The treatment has to be carried out at least three times, at one-week intervals, to make certain that the young mites are also destroyed. Good care and feeding are also important to strengthen the cat's condition. For a severe infestation the veterinarian will give the cat one or two injections that contain a miticidal preparation. Rub ointment into the affected areas daily, carefully removing the crusts as you do.

Toxoplasmosis

This disease is produced by one-celled animals (*Toxoplasma gondii*). Almost all mammals, birds, reptiles, and humans serve as intermediate hosts for this parasite. Only the cat excretes egglike permanent forms of the pathogen (oocysts) in its stool after an infection. In all other animal species and in humans, cysts of the pathogen settle in the body tissue and remain there.

After recovery from an infection, humans and animals are immune to toxoplasmosis pathogens.

Infestation: Cats can become infected through the oocysts in feces and by eating cyst-containing raw or undercooked meat (pork, goat, mutton) and infected prey (mice).

Symptoms and effects: In healthy adult cats toxoplasmosis

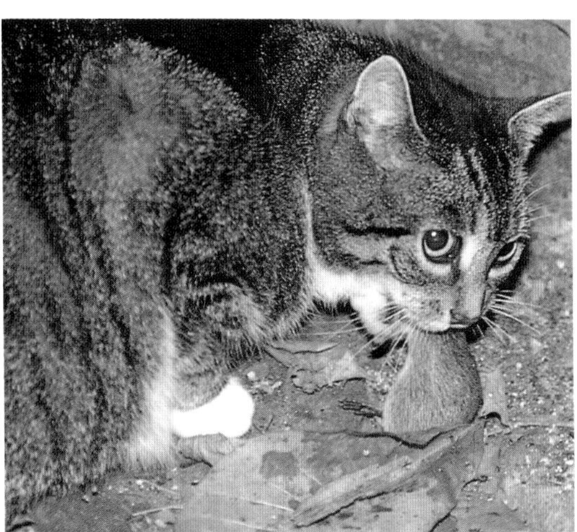

Mice frequently transmit the toxoplasmosis pathogen to cats. Young cats, can die of toxoplasmosis.

usually runs its course undetected. Apart from mild diarrhea it is asymptomatic. Especially in young cats, however, massive infections can give rise to general ill health, difficulty in breathing, coughing, diarrhea, jaundice, or paralysis. Very young cats sometimes die.

Risk to humans: Humans can become infected through the oocysts in cat's feces, or by eating raw or undercooked meat containing cysts. Raw meat is by far the most common source of infection for humans. The pathogens are destroyed by cooking, roasting, or deep-freezing.

Pregnant women in particular are often advised to get rid of their cats in order to eliminate the threat posed by cat feces. In an initial infection the toxoplasmosis pathogens can cause miscarriage or damage to the fetus. Getting rid of the cat, however, is not always justified. Most people are immune to toxoplasmosis because they have already recovered from an infection and have enough antibodies. For this reason women who are pregnant should first be tested by their physician to determine whether they have already had toxoplasmosis.

In addition, an indoor cat that is not fed uncooked meat is not likely to be a source of infection. If a stool test reveals that the cat is excreting oocysts, there is no cause for panic. Oocysts are excreted for only seven to 14 days after infection in a cat. If all the rules of good hygiene are followed and the stool is removed from the litter pan immediately (wear rubber gloves!), the danger of contagion is small. Pregnant women should discuss all their options with their obstetrician and their cat's veterinarian before giving their pet away.

● **Treatment**

▶ Proof of oocysts in a cat's stool is obtained by the veterinarian by means of the flotation procedure (see "Glossary," page 113). Serologic procedures can also be used with cats to provide evidence that infection has already taken place. Only live pathogens in the intestines can be treated with sulfonamides (see "Glossary" page 113).

Follow-up care: Sulfonamides for two to three weeks.

Prevention: Impossible with outdoor cats. Don't feed uncooked meat to indoor cats.

Cat Fleas

Male cat fleas are about 2.5 millimeters long, female fleas, 3.5 millimeters. Both have a brownish black chitinous exoskeleton. Their sides are flattened, and their rear legs have a great deal of spring. Fleas pierce the cat's skin and suck its blood. Then they excrete blood, only partially digested, in the form of comma-shaped crumblets of feces.

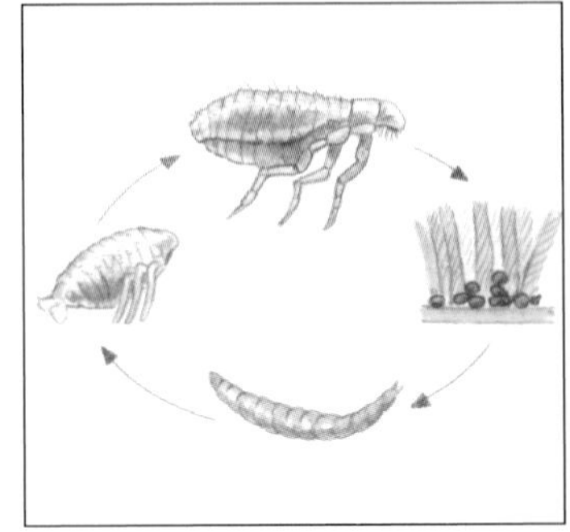

Developmental cycle of the cat flea: Fleas develop from the eggs in the cat's fur that fall to the ground, and the larvae live on flea dirt (dried blood).

Female fleas lay 20 to 30 eggs daily. The sticky eggs cling to the cat's coat but fall off as time passes. Larvae hatch from the eggs four to fourteen days after being laid. The mature larva pupates in a cocoon and changes into a young flea.

The developmental cycle of cat fleas can end after only 20 days, but sometimes it lasts as long as a year. The flea population is largest in late summer.

Infestation: Through direct contact between cats; at flea nests (nidi); dogs and humans can also be carriers.

Detection: With the naked eye, when combing through the coat with a fine-toothed flea comb (see drawing, page 23). Detection is also possible as follows: Lay what you believe to be crumblets of feces on a paper tissue and add a few drops of water. If a reddish brown ring forms around the crumblets, they are flea droppings (hemolyzed cat blood).

Effects: Frequently flea allergies, which can lead to severe skin inflammations (see "Disorders of the Skin and the Hormonal Glands," page 74). In a massive infestation the loss of blood can seriously weaken an adult cat. In young cats it can cause anemia (see page 95) and result in death. Fleas also function as intermediate hosts for tapeworms (see page 102).

Risk to humans: Cat fleas attack humans temporarily and cause itching.

● **Treatment**

- Once a week, treat the cat with an insecticidal powder (insecticide, see "Glossary," page 113). Adult cats may also be treated with a liquid flea insecticide that is dripped onto the coat, where it penetrates the skin. Consult with your veterinarian regarding which products and procedures are recommended for your area.
- Clean your cat's environment thoroughly, and wash blankets and cat beds. Disinfect the area with special sprays that kill flea larvae (available from the veterinarian or in pet stores).

Prevention: Many different products are available; your veterinarian can advise you as to what is best for your pet. Flea collars (available in pet stores) may be used on cats that are allowed outside. The collars emit insecticides for three to four months but have their drawbacks: the cat is in constant contact with poison, and a cat can strangle on the collar if the cat becomes caught somewhere. Check your pet regularly with a flea comb.

■ **Homeopathy**

See page 78.

Biting Lice

Biting lice, like fleas, are classified as insects. With a body length of 1.3 millimeters, the light-yellow cat lice are barely half the size of the brownish black fleas. Biting lice do not puncture the skin of their host to suck blood. They are content with skin scales and secretions flowing from scratches, which they ingest with the aid of their broad jaws. The biting louse passes through three larval stages of development. Biting lice stick their eggs one by one to the hairs of their host. If they are separated from "their cat," biting lice perish within 14 days. In contrast to the flea, the entire life cycle of the biting louse takes place on the cat.

Infestation: From one animal to another, rarely through grooming utensils (brush, comb). Primarily poorly groomed, weakened cats are endangered. Humans are not affected.

Detection: With the naked eye; plucked-out coat hairs or biting lice that have been combed out of the coat can be identified with a magnifying glass.

Effects: Skin damage resulting from scratching and nibbling. Hair loss, eczema, and infections can occur as consecutive symptoms if the infestation is severe. Biting lice can function as intermediate hosts for tapeworms (see page 102).

● **Treatment**

Treat affected animals several times, at ten-day intervals, with insecticidal powder.

Prevention: Flea collar (see "Cat Fleas," page 98), regular grooming. Consult your veterinarian regarding other treatment regimes.

■ **Homeopathy**

See page 78.

Ticks

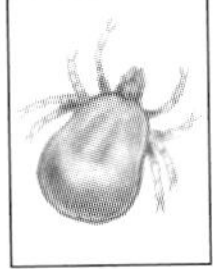

Cats are affected primarily by the common wood tick and by other scale ticks. As a tick develops it passes through a larval stage to the nymph stage and finally becomes a fully grown adult.

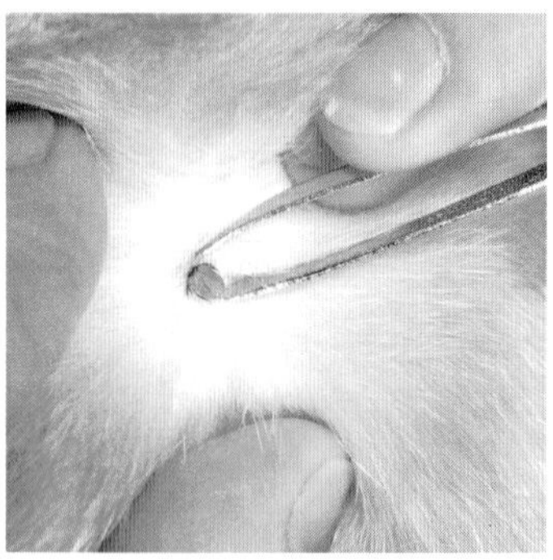

To remove a tick, grasp it with tweezers and rotate it.

Although the inconspicuous larvae are barely 1 millimeter long, mature female ticks that have sucked themselves full can attain a body length of over .4 inch (1 cm) and a weight of almost .0176 ounce (0.5 g). The large, plump females develop approximately 3,000 eggs, which grow in a sheltered place on the ground into a new generation of larvae. All the developmental stages of the tick search out animals whose blood they can suck.

Infestation: Especially in spring and fall ticks drop from plant stems or bushes onto cats and bore their way into the cats' skin. They cling there until they have sucked themselves full of blood (three to fourteen days). Only then does the tick drop off the cat. Cats are used as hosts chiefly by nymphs and adult ticks.

Detection: Ticks are found predominantly on the neck and head. They can be as large as pinheads or—when full of sucked blood—as large as peas (see photo, left).

Effects: The tick's site on the cat's skin can become inflamed and serve as a starting point for bacterial infections.

Risk to humans: Ticks also attack humans. Special kinds can carry borreliosis (see "Glossary," page 113) or Lyme disease, as well as viruses that cause meningitis.

● **Treatment**

Ticks are best removed with special tick tweezers (available in pet stores). Rotate the tweezers in any direction you choose. If the tick's head tears off, which happens in isolated instances, a skin inflammation results, although it rarely assumes serious proportions. In case of doubt consult the veterinarian. If the infestation is severe, the cat can be treated with insecticides.

Hint: Many people recommend dabbing oil or nail polish on the tick before removing it. According to the latest findings, that is inadvisable. It causes the tick to regurgitate its contents, which often include pathogens, into the wound.

Prevention: Check your cat's coat regularly if the cat is allowed outdoors; use tick collars (available in pet stores) that give off insecticides (see "Cat Fleas," page 98).

■ **Homeopathy**

See page 78.

Internal Parasites

Worms, which are classified as endoparasites (see "Glossary," page 113), occur in the cat's intestines and other organs. The three main types of internal parasites that thrive in the cat are *nematodes,* which resemble earthworms and include roundworms and hookworms; *protozoa,* which usually are one-celled organisms that contain specialized structures for feeding and locomotion; and *cestodes* (or tapeworms), which are carried by fleas.

Roundworms

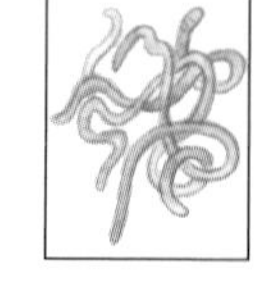

Roundworms (ascarids) live in the cat's small intestine and feed on intestinal contents. Female worms can reach a length of 4 inches (10 cm). They continually produce a large number of eggs, which can be excreted in the cat's stool. Roundworms require no intermediate hosts.

Contagion: Occurs either by picking up eggs through contact with infected feces or by ingesting eggs in infected prey or raw meat. Within four weeks larvae develop in the extremely hardy roundworm eggs. If a cat ingests the eggs, the larvae are released in its intestine. Some larvae bore through the intestinal wall and travel in the bloodstream into the lungs and from there into the trachea. The larvae are coughed upward, swallowed, and land back in the intestine, where they develop into adult roundworms. Larvae also can be encapsulated for years in the cat's muscles without causing any problems. Once the cat becomes pregnant, the larvae resume their activity, make their way into the cat's teats, and reach the intestines of newborn kittens in their mother's milk.

Symptoms and effects: A mild infestation of roundworms, commonly found in cats, produces no conspicuous symptoms. Occasionally roundworms are vomited up or eliminated in diarrhea. Cats with a severe infestation frequently have an intestinal inflammation accompanied by diarrhea; they lose weight, eat poorly, and have a dull coat. Intestinal obstruction (see page 87) and penetration of the worms into the abdominal cavity are rare.

Risk to humans: Occasionally, humans also become infected with larvae through infectious roundworm eggs. At greatest risk are children who play in sandboxes and come into contact with buried cat droppings. The infestation usually is asymptomatic. The infection can be determined by blood tests.

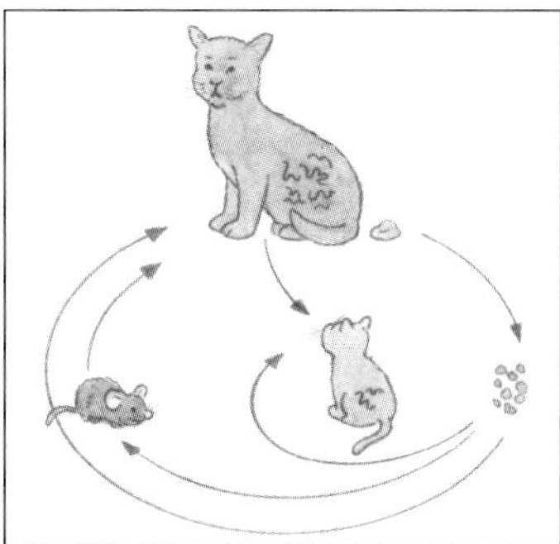

The roundworm cycle: Adult cats are infected primarily by roundworm eggs. A roundworm infection is transmitted to young kittens through their mother's milk.

- **Treatment**

▶ Your veterinarian will examine a fecal sample under a microscope. There are several agents that are effective against roundworms, and they are well tolerated by cats.

Follow-up care: Deworming agents are available from veterinarians. To learn how to administer them, see illustration, page 27. Deworm kittens according to the schedule on page 27. Deworm older cats once or twice a year, depending on their risk of infection.

It is advisable that your veterinarian periodically examine your pet's stool under a microscope to monitor any infestation and the success of the treatment.

Prevention: Impossible with outdoor cats. With indoor cats always remove fresh feces from the litter pan at once, as roundworm eggs need about four weeks to become infectious.

Hookworms

Adult hookworms live in the cat's small intestine. They subsist on intestinal mucosa and suck blood. In moderate climates however, hookworm infestations are less common than are roundworm infestations.

Contagion: The thin-shelled hookworm eggs leave the body of an infected cat in its stool. The hatching larvae develop best at high ambient temperatures and in humidity. The infectious larvae can actively penetrate into an animal through its skin or mucous membranes, or eggs may be ingested. Hookworm larvae migrate through the cat's body and, just like roundworms, can infect newborn kittens through their mother's milk.

Symptoms and effects: Cats severely infested with hookworms suffer from diarrhea, which frequently contains blood and mucus. Their coats become dull, and they grow thin and weak. The constant loss of blood (a single hookworm consumes 0.1 milliliter daily) results in anemia (see page 95). Young cats in particular can die of anemia.

Risk to humans: Hookworm larvae can pierce the skin. Usually only skin reactions result, in rare instances lung diseases and bronchitis. Children who play bare-armed and bare-legged in damp places run the greatest risk of infection.

● Treatment

▶ Microscopic evidence of the thin-shelled oval eggs is obtained by means of fecal flotation (see "Glossary," page 113). The veterinarian will prescribe anthelmintics (see "Glossary," page 113), which the owner usually can give the cat by mouth. In addition, weakened, anemic cats need to be given supplementary iron, minerals, and protein.

Stomach Worms

The feline stomach worm is only 1 millimeter long. Common worldwide, it also affects other small- and large-cat species, sometimes even foxes, dogs, and pigs. The diminutive worms live concealed in the gastric mucosa.

Contagion: The worms multiply in the cat's stomach. They frequently cause vomiting in affected animals, and worms and larvae leave the cat's body in each vomitus. A new host becomes infected when it eats the regurgitated stomach contents. Stray cats in particular gladly accept this "food supply."

Symptoms and effects: Usually the infestation causes no detectable symptoms other than more-frequent vomiting. If the infestation is severe, inflammation of the gastric mucosa (see page 86) can also lead to corresponding symptoms.

Tapeworms

Tapeworms live in the cat's small intestine. They require at least one intermediate host (for example, fleas, mice, or rats) for their development. If the cat catches an infected mouse, the tapeworm develops into its sexually mature form in the cat's intestines. The ripe, egg-filled terminal segments are continuously cast off by the tapeworm, leaving the cat's body with its stool. When a mouse eats these tapeworm segments or ingests food contaminated by eggs, it becomes infected.

● Treatment

▶ If a suspicion exists, only a microscopic examination of prepared regurgitated gastric contents can supply proof.

Levamisol and Oxfendazol are said to be effective anthelmintics (see "Glossary," page 113).

Lung Worms

The lung worm is a nematode that lives in the lungs of infected cats. By the time they have reached the adult stage, lung worms are threaded through the tissue of the cat's lungs. The female worm lays eggs that develop and hatch in the lung. The resulting larvae migrate up the trachea and enter the digestive tract by way of the esophagus.

Contagion: The process by which lung worms infect a cat is a complex one. Lung worm larvae do not set up housekeeping in the cat's gut. Instead, the larvae are passed into the external environment via the cat's feces. Unless the larvae are eaten by a snail or a slug, they never can develop into a stage in which they are able to infect a cat. If they are eaten by a snail, however, lung worm larvae will migrate to the snail's body tissues, where the larvae evolve into an infective stage.

Next, a small rodent has to eat the infected snail or slug. After that, the lung worm larvae turn into cysts in the tissues of the rodent. Finally, a cat has to eat the infected rodent or snail.

Symptoms and effects: Lung worms generally produce the symptoms of mild respiratory distress. In critical cases the signs of distress are more pronounced, and the cat's breathing might be affected to an extent that could cause death.

● Treatment

▶ The presence of lung worms is indicated by the presence of the larval stage of the worm in the cat's feces. Cats infected with lung worms should be treated with worming medications.

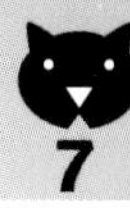

Cat Tapeworm

The cat tapeworm is the most common of the tapeworms that affect cats. It grows in the small intestine to a length of up to 24 inches (60 cm). A cat can have several tapeworms at the same time.

Contagion: Cats that are allowed outdoors become infected primarily through their prey, the mouse, which in turn can become infected via the cat's feces.

Symptoms and effects: Whitish tapeworm segments, flexible at first and the size of a grain of rice, are present in the cat's stool or in its coat near the anus. Usually no discernible symptoms are present in the cat itself, but massively infested young cats can be delayed in their development, have a dull coat, lack appetite, and lose weight.

Risk to humans: Rare, isolated cases have been described in which a human also has become infected with cat tapeworm eggs through cat feces.

● Treatment

▶ As a rule the veterinarian will recommend treatment with the active substance Praziquantel (see "Glossary," page 113). This drug is the most effective means of controlling all the types of tapeworms that occur in cats. Even if the tapeworm has been destroyed, a free roaming cat can become reinfected shortly following the treatment by ingesting another intermediate host. After several weeks the reinfected cat will again pass tapeworm segments in its stool.

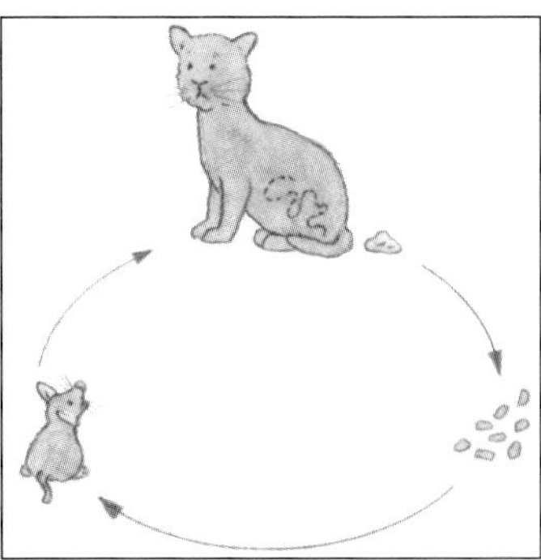

The tapeworm cycle: The cat tapeworm is generally transmitted by mice. The cat eliminates the tapeworm segments, which resemble grains of rice, in its stool.

Prevention: Cats that are not allowed outside are well protected against the cat tapeworm.

Infectious Diseases

By "infectious diseases" we mean diseases that are caused by microorganisms such as viruses, bacteria, and fungi. These diseases are highly contagious as a rule. Fortunately, vaccines for the prevention of many dangerous infectious diseases are available today. Consequently, all responsible cat owners must have their pets vaccinated as a preventive measure and must have the appropriate booster shots given on schedule (see "Vaccination Schedule for Preventive Health Care" page 26).

Feline Infectious Peritonitis (FIP)

Symptoms: Fever, refusal to eat, weight loss, apathy, diarrhea, vomiting, dehydration, paralysis, difficulty breathing, large abdomen.

Causes and effects: A coronavirus produces this disease. Although the overwhelming majority of cats (if not all cats) are affected by an infection of this kind, only a few fall ill and die of FIP. In recent years a great deal of research has been done on this disease. Nevertheless, it continues to be one of the most mysterious and dreaded diseases of cats. We know, for example, that stressful situations can trigger FIP in a cat. Weeks, months, or years may pass between the time of infection and the outbreak of the disease (initial symptoms). The details of the paths of infection, the incubation period, and the course of the disease are still unclear.

The outbreak of the disease is insidious at first; it typically leads to an accumulation of fluid (ascites) in the cat's abdominal cavity. According to recent findings, this is not, as first suspected, attributable to peritonitis but to a general inflammation and impairment of small blood vessels.

In addition, other manifestations of this disease frequently occur in which, for example, predominantly the chest cavity, intestines, or central nervous system are affected and no ascites are present. Once the disease has broken out, it progresses steadily and is almost always fatal.

- **Treatment**

► The typical manifestation involving ascites can be diagnosed by the veterinarian through examination. For atypical forms, which are becoming increasingly common, there is as yet no lab test suited for use in a veterinary office laboratory.

Once the disease has broken out, there is no promising therapy. Only the discomfort can be

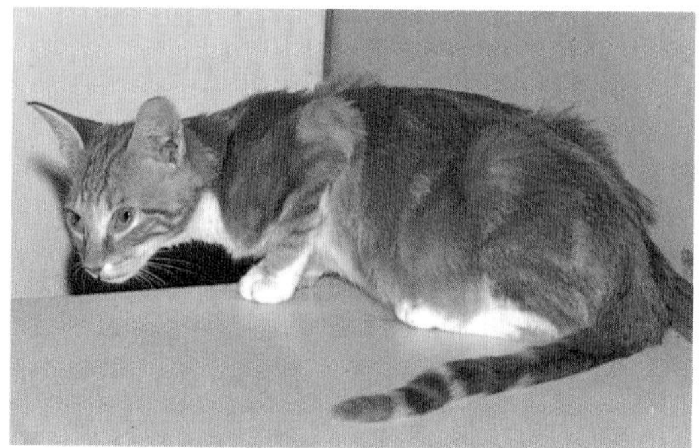

This cat is suffering from FIP in the advanced stage. It is emaciated, and its behavior is apathetic.

relieved initially with medications. Because FIP is an immune disease, cortisone treatments, among other things, have been tried, but without convincing success. Recurring reports of cures through homeopathy should be regarded with some skepticism. If the disease develops to the point that the cat is suffering considerably (for example, it has difficulty breathing) or becomes completely apathetic, you should have it put to sleep painlessly.

Prevention: If an indoor cat has died of FIP, you should have your home (cushions, wall-to-wall carpet, the cat's favorite spots) thoroughly cleaned and then disinfected. Wait at least three to four weeks before bringing a new cat home. It takes that long for the danger of infection to disappear.

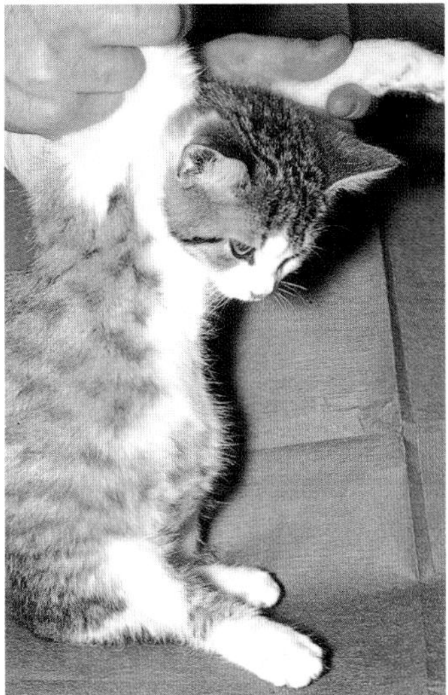

An accumulation of fluid in the abdominal area (ascites) is typical of FIP infection.

Several factors promote the outbreak of FIP. Make sure that:

- you don't have too many cats living in too small a space (stress)
- you provide optimum living conditions and care
- a cat suffering from FIP is kept isolated from healthy cats

Vaccination: Since 1991 an FIP vaccine has been used successfully in the United States. The ideal time for the first vaccination is the kitten's sixteenth week of life.

The vaccination is repeated after three weeks and booster shots are given every twelve months. Unfortunately, this vaccination cannot help acutely ill cats.

Aujeszky's Disease (Pseudorabies)

Symptoms: See "Rabies," page 108; severe itching; instances of sudden death.

Causes and effects: This disease, caused by a herpes virus, occurs primarily among pigs, which frequently harbor the virus without becoming ill. Thus, it is possible for pork to contain infectious viruses, despite official inspections of meat and animals for slaughter. The disease is also transmissible to rats, dogs, cats, and several other animal species. In a typical case the disease in cats produces rabies-like manifestations, and severe itching is frequently present as well. Death can occur very quickly, however, even without symptoms of this kind.

Risk to humans: The virus is not dangerous. It is killed by cooking meat.

- **Treatment**

▶ Infected animals are beyond help.

Prevention: Never feed a cat raw or half-cooked pork (cooking kills the pathogen).

Vaccination: Although the vaccine used with pigs could also safeguard cats and dogs, it is not approved for use with those species.

Pox Virus Infection

Pox virus infection in cats was first described in 1980. Several cases have been recorded since that time.

Symptoms: The disease causes pustules and ulcers, primarily on the head but also on the feet and sometimes over the entire body. Complications are produced by bacteria and by fungal infections.

Causes and effects: An animal pox virus, probably identical to the cowpox virus that attacks rodents. Cats are infected by their prey.

FeLV—a Dangerous Viral Infection

Feline leukemia virus (FeLV) disease is the term used for a tumorous disorder of the blood-forming and lymphatic tissues. FeLV is an infectious disease that is common worldwide and affects many animals.

Symptoms: Lack of appetite, diarrhea, increased thirst, fever, weight loss, difficulty breathing, swollen lymph nodes, pale mucous membranes, increases in girth, abnormal behavior.

Causes and effects: Generally, FeLV (the feline leukemia virus) is responsible for causing leukemia and related diseases in cats. It belongs to the family of retroviruses. Cats can become infected through close physical contact with others of their kind (bites, licking, mating). The virus can also be passed on to unborn kittens in the womb of a pregnant cat. The incubation period is several weeks, months, or even years. Not all cats that are infected actually develop the FeLV disease. The immune system of a cat with a good constitution frequently is able to destroy the virus. If the disease breaks out, however, it can appear in a great many guises. First the bone marrow suffers damage, which often shows up in the form of changes in the blood count and anemia (see page 95). Finally, tumors, nerve damage, and fertility disorders can appear. Many secondary consequences of the FeLV disease result from suppression of the body's immune system (immune suppression, see "Glossary," page 113). Affected cats become susceptible to other infections. Some cats harbor the viruses in their blood for a very long time and can pass on the infection without developing symptoms themselves (latent virus shedders).

Risk to other animal species and to humans: Although feline leukemia viruses grow on cell cultures that come from other animal species and from humans as well, it has never been possible to prove that a transmission of the disease occurred.

● **Treatment**

▶ If there are grounds for suspicion, see a veterinarian immediately. The presence of the virus in blood or saliva is certain evidence of infection. This detection is now being made with standard veterinary diagnostic tests. Once a cat owner notices the symptoms described above in his or her pet, the disease often is already well under way. As a rule the cat is already beyond all help, and death comes very quickly. If the symptoms are mild or if the infected animal is asymptomatic, an attempt can be made to strengthen the cat's natural resistance with medications called paramunity inducers (see "Glossary," page 113).

Vaccination: Vaccines that render a cat immune to the FeLV disease have been available for several years. As a rule, however, before the first vaccination is given a test must be made to ascertain whether the cat has already been affected by feline leukemia viruses. Acutely diseased animals cannot be protected by vaccination.

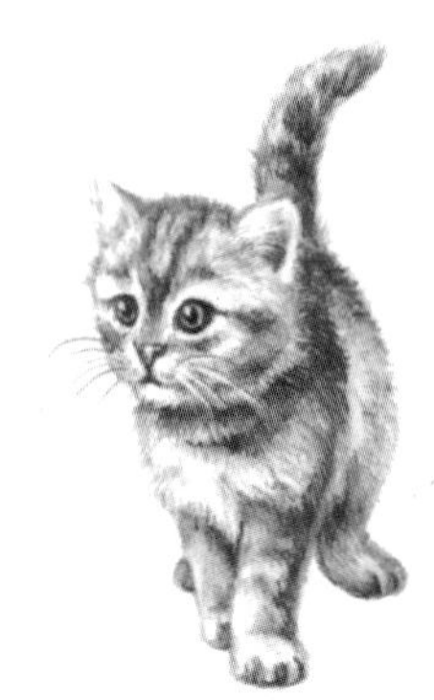

Risk to humans: Many people no longer have immunity to small pox because the disease has died out. Consequently they can become infected with the animal pox virus. At greatest risk are children, the elderly, and people with weakened immune systems. Infection with animal pox virus via cats, however, has not thus far attained any significance.

- **Treatment**

▶ Only the vet can tell whether your cat is actually infected with the virus. No treatment is possible. Spontaneous healing occurs after a few weeks, but occasionally there are fatal forms.

Feline Panleukopenia (Parvovirus Disease)

Symptoms: Apathy, watery or bloody diarrhea, vomiting, high fever, stomachache (animal cries out in pain when touched).

Causes and effects: Feline panleukopenia (FPL, parvovirus disease) is caused by parvoviruses. The FPL viruses are highly resistant and capable of remaining contagious for over a year at normal ambient temperatures. Consequently, cats become ill not only through direct contact with diseased cats but also through mediators and virus-contaminated objects (toys, coat-grooming utensils, food bowls). The interval between infection and the outbreak of the disease (incubation period) is roughly two to 10 days.

Feline panleukopenia is usually accompanied by a painful inflammation of the intestines. In the course of the disease the number of white corpuscles drops sharply, which results in lowered resistance. Bacterial infections then can develop unhindered.

Frequently, FPL leads to death so quickly that one might suspect poisoning. Young cats in particular sometimes die before any symptoms are noticed. If pregnant cats become ill, their offspring can be impaired.

- **Treatment**

▶ If there are grounds for suspicion, see a veterinarian at once. In young cats and unvaccinated cats FPL can be assumed on the basis of the symptoms. Intensive treatment has to be started at once. Lab tests will confirm the diagnosis. To compensate for the loss of fluids and electrolytes (see "Glossary," page 113), the cat first will be given infusions. Antibiotics are used to combat secondary bacterial infections. The veterinarian will give the cat analgesics, antispasmodics, and antiemetics. Hyperimmune serums (passive immunization) may also be employed to block free virus particles.

Follow-up care: If the cat is not kept in an animal hospital, it needs intensive care on a twenty-four-hour basis if it is to have any chance of survival. Daily infusions by the veterinarian are required.

Vaccination: Effective vaccines (see "Vaccination Schedule for Preventive Health Care," page 26) to prevent feline panleukopenia have long been available. Pregnant cats should not be inoculated with the live vaccine because damage to the kittens cannot be ruled out.

Feline Respiratory Disease

Symptoms: Harmless forms progress with occasional sneezing. In severe forms, watery to purulent nasal discharge, impairment of mucous membranes, watering eyes, conjunctivitis, coughing, drooling, difficulty breathing, refusal to eat, dehydration, apathy.

Causes: The so-called "cat flu" or "cat cold" is not a uniform disease. Several types of viruses and bacterial pathogens can cause respiratory disease in cats. The most severe forms of the disease are caused by caliciviruses and herpes viruses. Other viruses (retroviruses, for example), chlamydia, and various bacteria can produce similar, usually fairly harmless diseases and/or complicate the existing illness.

Stress situations, particularly those resulting from keeping too many cats in too small an area (pet shelters, boarding catteries, breeders), promote a serious course of the disease.

Effects: With severe forms frequent developments include inflammation of the oral mucous membranes, bronchitis, and inflammations of the lung. Cats that refuse to eat and become dehydrated often die of debilitation.

● **Treatment**

▶ See a veterinarian at the first signs of illness. Special tests are required to identify the pathogens precisely. If the cat is already seriously dehydrated, it will be given infusions to compensate for the loss of electrolytes and nutrients. Antibiotics are used to fight bacteria and chlamydia. If the mucous membranes are damaged, the cat is given anti-inflammatories. The use of hyperimmune serum (see "Glossary," page 113) has also proved helpful in many cases.

Follow-up care: It is important to nurse the cat back to health in familiar surroundings with a great deal of devotion (see page 50). At this time a cat needs a warm bed and hygienic conditions. Using a paper tissue dipped in chamomile solution, clean encrusted nostrils regularly. Inhalations can alleviate the discomfort. Prepare a chamomile infusion, place the cat in a pet carrier that can be latched, and set the chamomile infusion in a bowl in front of the carrier. With a cloth, fan the hot chamomile vapors into the carrier so that the cat inhales them.

Prevention: Optimum environmental and living conditions.

Vaccination: Reliable vaccines to prevent the most dangerous viruses (calici and herpes) have been available for years. The cat can also be vaccinated against chlamydia bacteria, which on their own cause rather harmless but protracted diseases.

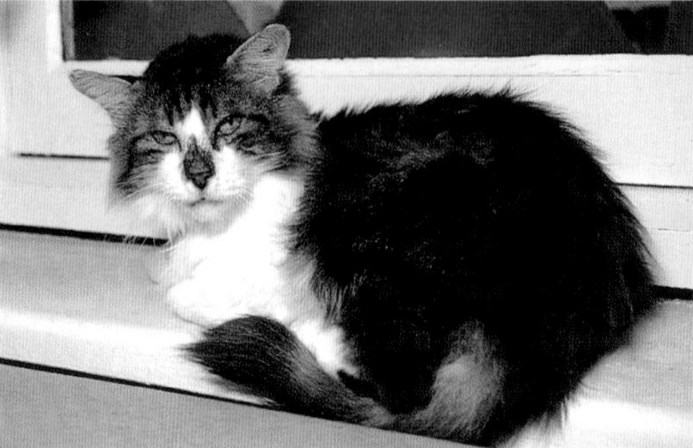

Feline respiratory disease is not a uniform disease. Several types of viruses and bacterial pathogens can cause "colds" in cats.

Rabies

Symptoms: Lack of appetite, weight loss, abnormal behavior.

Causes and effects: The rabies virus belongs to the rhabdovirus family. Mammals, birds, and humans can contract rabies (zoonosis, see "Glossary," page 113). Rabies viruses are excreted in the saliva of diseased animals and usually are transmitted to other animals and humans through a bite. It is also possible for the viruses to penetrate through wounds or mucous membranes. After an incubation period of fourteen days to two months, during which the viruses multiply and advance along the nerve paths to reach the brain, the first symptoms appear. The destruction of the nerve cells results in manifestations of restlessness, behavioral changes, and, finally, paralysis before death occurs.

Rabies has three phases. First, the cat's customary behavior changes. It may be, for example, shy, fearful, and restless, or precisely the opposite—exceptionally tame and affectionate. In the second phase the cat drools heavily, has convulsions, and is aggressive. After the third phase—the paralysis stage—the cat dies. Rabies does not always progress in this typical form, however.

Risk to humans: Rabies viruses are communicable to humans. For our protection and peace of mind the domestic animals with which we live in close contact should be vaccinated against rabies. Even immediately after a possible infection, humans can be protected by immunization against the outbreak of the disease.

- **Treatment**

▶ If there are grounds for suspicion, go to a veterinarian at once. Treatment is futile and also prohibited because of the threat posed by a rabid animal.

Safety precautions must be taken without delay for the protection of humans and other animals. The suspicion has to be reported to the appropriate veterinary authorities (Reportable Zoonosis). Only special tests performed on its brain after the animal's death make an accurate diagnosis possible.

Vaccination: Reliable vaccines have been available for years. If used regularly, they provide protection against rabies. A cat that is kept indoors at all times has no risk of infection and, therefore, theoretically does not need to be vaccinated, but if the pet is scheduled to attend shows or to travel abroad, legal regulations may require vaccination. What's more, indoor cats that slip outdoors can become infected if they have not been vaccinated.

Feline Immune Deficiency Virus (FIV, Feline AIDS)

Symptoms: No specific indications. Many affected cats first suffer from the symptoms of feline respiratory disease (see page 107).

Cause and effects: The feline immunodeficiency virus (FIV), very closely related to the human immunodeficiency virus, is a member of the retrovirus family. The virus is transmitted from one cat to another via saliva and blood, probably largely through a bite. The virus multiplies in the immune cells of the infected cat, destroying them. In that way viruses, bacteria, or parasites are able to develop unchecked and cause many different diseases. Many chronic infections of various organ systems, including chronic gingivitis, for example, can be caused by a weakened immune system.

Risk to humans: As far as we know at this time, the virus cannot be transmitted by cats to humans.

- **Treatment**

▶ A veterinarian can detect FIV antibodies on the basis of a serologic test of the cat's blood.

In diseased animals the secondary diseases are treated in order to improve the cat's condition temporarily.

Prevention: Stray cats are predominantly affected by the virus. Indoor cats with no opportunity to be with stray cats are safe from infection.

Vaccination: Unfortunately, there is as yet no vaccine against FIV.

Tetanus (Lockjaw)

The tetanus pathogens (*Clostridium tetani*) make their way into open wounds and form spores (permanent forms). They excrete a poison that attacks the cat's nerves and causes cramping in all its muscles.

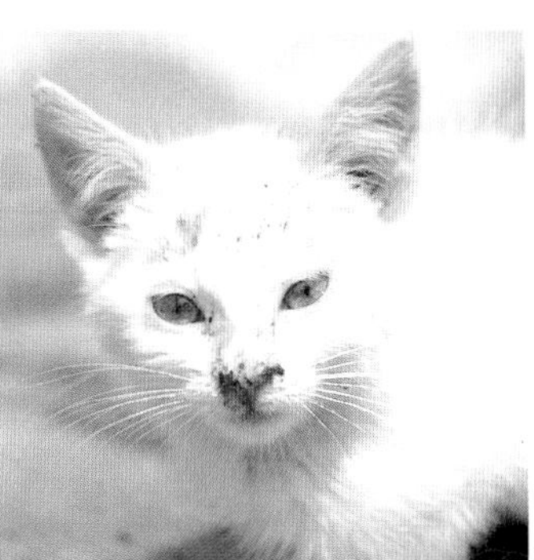

FIV (feline AIDS) has no clear-cut symptoms. Many cats with this disease first display symptoms of feline respiratory disease, such as nasal discharge or conjunctivitis.

Symptoms and effects: Affected cats suffer at first from a cramping of the facial muscles, until the poisons have spread via the nerve paths in the spine and the brain. Then all the muscles are affected by spasms. There is heavy drooling because the cat no longer can swallow. In the advanced stage high fever is usual. Frequently the affected cat dies.

Causes: Transmission of tetanus pathogens by dirt that gets into a wound (for example, through accidents, bites, insect stings).

● **Treatment**

▶ Possible only by a veterinarian. Although the tetanus pathogens can be successfully destroyed by penicillin, the devastating effect of the poison in the body continues. Antitoxins have to be injected. In addition, the cat will be given antispasmodic sedatives. Usually the cat's chances of survival are poor.

Vaccination: Cats are at less risk from tetanus than are humans. Vaccination against tetanus is certainly possible but not usual. A veterinarian will suggest a tetanus vaccination only if the cat has extremely dangerous wounds.

Bacterial Infections

Diseases that are caused by bacteria frequently develop in cats after a viral infection. Unlike viruses, bacteria can be destroyed with antibiotics. Penicillin was the first antibiotic discovered for medical use. Not all types of bacteria can be controlled with the same medication, however. Some bacterial strains can also become resistant to previously effective agents.

Chlamydia and mycoplasms: These bacteria attack primarily the conjunctiva and the mucous membranes in the cat's head. Often, along with other pathogens, they produce a more or less distinct syndrome, which we have attributed to the "Feline Respiratory Disease" (see page 107). Tetracyclines are the drugs of choice to combat these bacteria.

Salmonella: Cats can be attacked by salmonella bacteria, which reside principally in the intestines and can cause diarrhea and serious systemic diseases. These bacteria also can live in a cat without producing symptoms, however. Then the animal will excrete salmonella without becoming ill itself. Humans acquire salmonella chiefly through contaminated or spoiled food. In people with lowered resistance serious illnesses result from salmonella. If a cat is found to have salmonella, appropriate precautionary measures are essential (for example, wearing rubber gloves when cleaning the cat's litter box). The medication Chloramphenicol is most often used against salmonella.

Coli bacteria: Coli bacteria usually live unobtrusively in the intestines, but under certain circumstances they can also cause diseases.

Pyogenic organisms (Staphylococci, streptococci): Pyogenic organisms frequently play a role in the formation of cat-bite abscesses.

Tuberculosis

This infectious disease, transmitted by the tubercle bacilli (*Mycobacterium tuberculosis*), rarely occurs in cats. There are three different types of mycobacteria, which cause diseases in humans, cattle, and birds. It is possible for tubercle bacilli to be transmitted by humans to cats.

Symptoms: Lack of appetite, weight loss, fatigue, shortness of breath, coughing, bouts of fever; in the advanced stage, diarrhea, vomiting, jaundice.

Cause and effects: Bacterial infection. In cats tuberculosis takes a chronic, "creeping" course and can attack all the tissues and organs.

Risk to humans: Tuberculosis bacteria are communicable by cats to humans.

● **Treatment**

▶ If tuberculosis has been detected in a cat, no therapy is initiated. The animal has to be put to sleep because of the danger of contagion it presents.

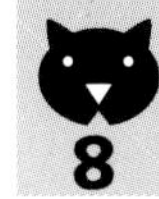

Pseudotuberculosis

Rarely, cats develop pseudotuberculosis, caused by infected prey.

Symptoms: See "Tuberculosis," page 110.

Cause and effects: Bacterial infection; the disease usually is fatal in cats.

Risk to humans: Cats can transmit the pathogens to humans.

● **Treatment**

▶ If there is proof that the cat has been attacked by the pathogens, prolonged treatment with medications theoretically can be initiated. Nevertheless, the disease usually proves fatal.

It is preferable to have the cat put to sleep, if only because of the danger of contagion for humans.

Fungal Infections

Fungi are classified as members of the vegetable kingdom. They grow in the form of filamentous elements (mycelium). They multiply and spread by means of extremely hardy spores. Some fungi use living organisms for their metabolic process.

Fungal diseases of the skin: Because of their symptoms they are the easiest to recognize (see "Disorders of the Skin and the Hormonal Glands," page 74) and also the most significant.

Systemic fungal diseases (see page 76): Far more rarely other tissues of the body are also affected by fungal infections. Because of their direct contact with the outside world, the principal candidates are the respiratory organs, mucous membranes, and intestinal tract. Fungal infections of such a general nature are very hard to diagnose, and they can give rise to life-threatening disease processes.

Owing to their rarity and uncharacteristic symptoms, systemic fungal infections (mycosis) frequently go undetected or are detected too late. Treatment with antifungal medications (Ketoconazol, Amphothericin B) is protracted.

Allergies: Mold fungi spores are especially likely to trigger allergies.

Fungal poisons: Some mold fungi that attack foodstuffs secrete toxins that can lead to symptoms of poisoning and, above all, to liver damage and tumors.

Risk to humans: Because fungi can also attack humans, strict precautionary measures have to be taken if your cat has a fungal infection. Your veterinarian will give you appropriate instructions.

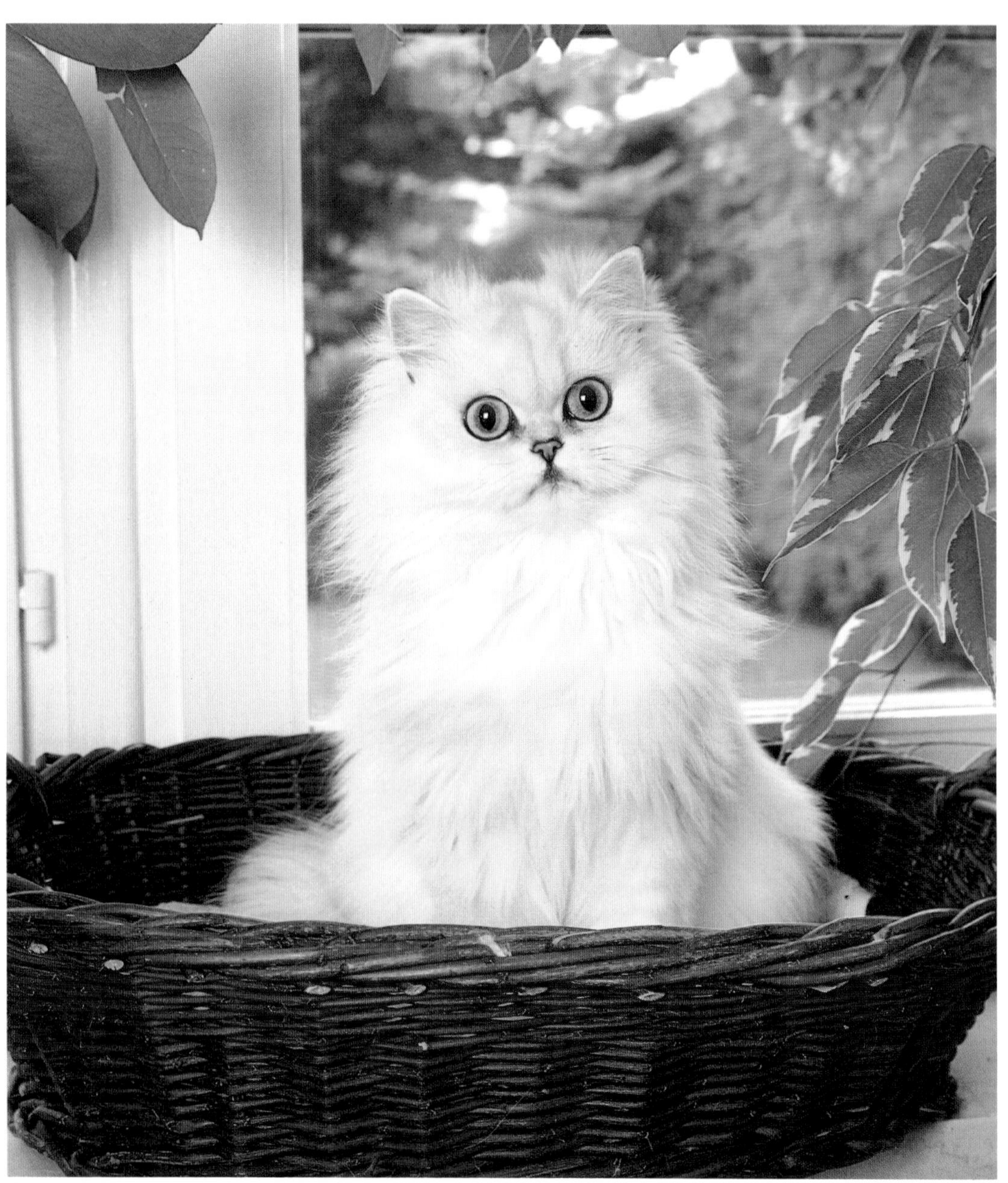

This chinchilla silver Persian cat, with its sea-green eyes, is a real beauty.

Glossary

In connection with the health—both good and ill—of their pets, cat owners often are confronted with technical terms that they are unable to make sense of at first. The professional terminology used by veterinarians, however, is not a sealed book. The most important concepts are explained in the following pages.

Aerosol
Medicine suitable for inhalation therapy; contains liquid substances dispersed in superfine form. Can indicate any particulate matter dispersed through air in superfine form—e.g. aerosolized viral particles.

Albino
Albus = white. Albino cats have few or no color pigments and, consequently, a snow-white coat, pale pink skin, and light-blue eyes with red pupils.

Allergens
Allergy-inducing substances.

Allergy
Abnormal, exaggerated reaction of the immune system to a substance, usually a protein, that is generally harmless.

Alopecia
Baldness.

Altering
Removal of the reproductive glands: in males, the testicles (castration), in females, the ovaries (spaying). Through altering, the sex drive and sexual behavior are eliminated, and the animals can no longer reproduce.

Analgesics
Remedies that allay or relieve pain.

Anemia
Reduced number of red blood cells or of hemoglobin within red blood cells.

Anthelmintics
Medicines that are effective against intestinal worms.

Antibiotics
Active substances that destroy bacteria or inhibit their growth.

Antibodies
Naturally existing antitoxins in the body that react with the antigen (pathogen) and render its harmless.

Antidote
Remedy to counteract the effects of poison.

Antiemetics
Remedies to inhibit vomiting.

Antimycotics
Remedies to control fungi.

Antiphlogistics
Anti-inflammatory drugs.

Apathy
Lack of interest.

Ascites
Increased accumulation of fluid in the abdominal cavity.

Atrophy of the kidney
End result of severe kidney disease.

Aujeszky's disease
Viral disease that is fatal to cats.

Autoimmune diseases
Diseases in which the body's natural tissue is destroyed by its own immune system.

Bacteria
Simple unicellular organisms that in some cases can cause diseases.

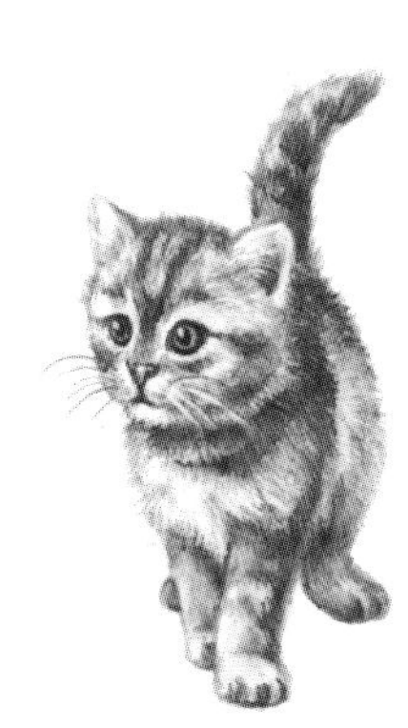

Bad breath
Cats can develop severe halitosis if they are fed fish, for example, but putrid breath also can be an indication of inflamed gums, abscessed teeth, or some other serious disease. The cat should be taken to a veterinarian.

Bezoars
Hair balls that are created in the stomach when the cat swallows hairs in the process of grooming its coat. Normally the animal regurgitates them again, but if it fails to do so, the bezoars can block the intestines. The results include constipation, apathetic behavior, vomiting, and loss of appetite. In less serious cases 1/2 teaspoonful of mineral oil or a commercial cat laxative will help. If no improvement is evident, the animal has to be taken to a veterinarian (see "Constipation," page 86).

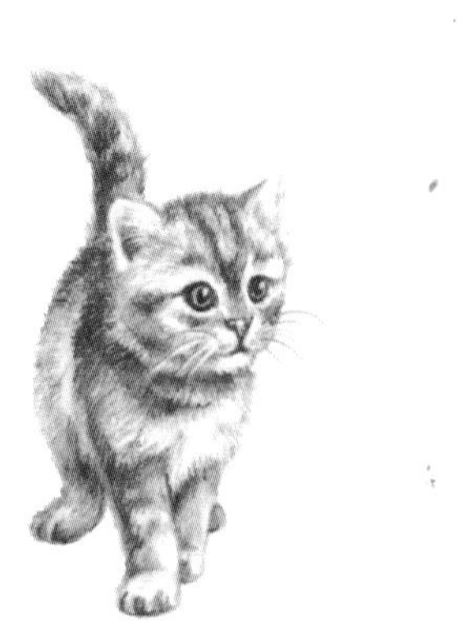

Biopsy
Removal of tissue sample by excision with a scalpel, puncture with a cannula, or in the process of endoscopy (see *Endoscopy*). Tissue samples are examined under a microscope.

Blood count
Analysis of the red and white blood corpuscles.

Blood plasma
Liquid portion of the blood in which blood cells are transported.

Blood values
Measured values of the substances dissolved in the blood—for example, blood sugar and urea—that have diagnostic significance.

Borreliosis
Infection transmitted by ticks.

Broad-spectrum antibiotic
Antibiotic effective against many types of bacteria.

C

Chlamydia
Special type of bacteria that can cause disease.

Chromosomes
Cats have 38 chromosomes, which carry the genes and are arranged in pairs in all the cells of the body. In female cats all pairs of chromosomes consist of two chromosomes that look alike. In male cats, however, one pair of chromosomes does not match one another. These are the male's sex chromosomes, and they determine the sex of his kittens.

Clinical examination
Determination of the state of health and/or the symptoms of disease by means of physical data and history that the veterinarian obtains by examination of the pet and consultation with the owner.

Complex preparations
Concept from homeopathy. Medications that contain several individual remedies with a similar effect.

Corticosteroids
Synthetic cortisones.

Cortisone
Hormone of the adrenal cortex that acts as an anti-inflammatory and has other effects as well.

Culture and sensitivity test
A test, performed on a culture containing a bacterial organism, that helps to identify the antibiotics to which the organism is sensitive.

D

Diagnosis
Process of determining the cause of a disease.

Digitalis glycosides
Medications, originally derived from foxglove (digitalis), which promote cardiac efficiency.

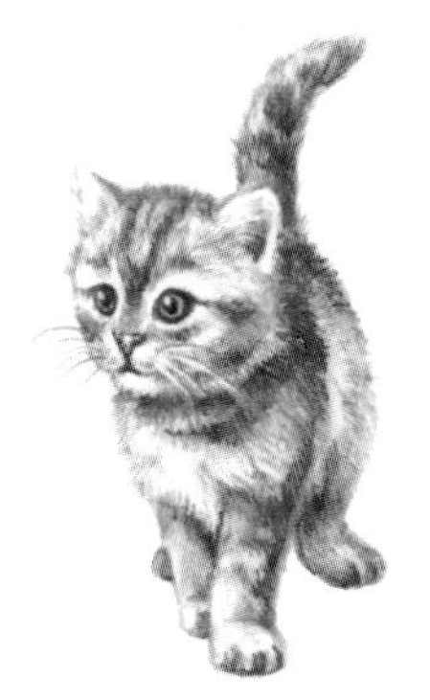

Diuretics
Agents that increase the volume of urine excreted.

Dysplasia
Abnormality of a tissue, usually congenital. For example, hip dysplasia.

Ectoparasites
External parasites such as fleas, mites, ticks, and lice.

Edema
Accumulation of fluid in various body tissues.

Electrocardiogram (ECG)
Detection and recording of electrical currents that originate during cardiac activity.

Electrolytes
Soluble salts and minerals (sodium, potassium, calcium, and magnesium, for example) important for bodily function and present in certain concentrations in the blood.

Elizabethan collar
In rare cases a cat wears an Elizabethan collar made of a stiff material after surgery to keep the cat from licking or chewing at the wound.

Endoparasites
Parasites that occur inside the body: e.g., worms.

Endoscopy
Observation of internal body cavities by means of a special fiberoptic instrument.

Enzymes
Substances produced in the living cell that influence the entire metabolic process in the body.

Extraction
Pulling out, of a tooth, for example.

Exudate
Substance exuded, e.g., purulent, crusty lesion of the skin.

Fatty liver
Increased storage of fat in the liver. Normal fat storage provides some protection against poisons because the fat stores the poisons and thus protects the liver cells. Too much fat, however, results in a constant strain on the organ. The result is a fatty degeneration of the liver.

Fecal flotation
See *Flotation*.

Fever
The cat's normal body temperature ranges from 100 to 103°F (37.8–39.2°C). A cat has fever only if its temperature is 103.1°F (39.3°C) or higher.

Flotation
Process for separating worm eggs from stool samples for diagnostic purposes.

Fungicides
Agents that kill fungi.

Gene
A biological unit containing an individual's genetic codes or traits.

Hair follicle
Small cavity from which a hair grows; it can become inflamed, for example, when acne (see page 75) is present.

Health insurance
For several years now insurance companies have also offered health insurance for cats. The type of coverage available varies with the insurance company. (See "Information," page 126.)

Hematoma
A localized swelling caused by effusion of blood into tissue.

Hereditary disease
Any disease passed on to subsequent generations through the genes (see *Inbreeding*).

Homeopathy
Method of treatment elevated to a principle 200 years ago. It involves the use of a series of dilutions of substances to combat symptoms of disease.

Hyperimmune serum
Blood serum that contains an extremely large number of specific antibodies. Used for therapy and derived from specially treated donor animals.

Icterus
Jaundice. The mucous membranes and skin turn yellow from increased bile pigments in the blood. Appears primarily with liver damage.

Immune deficiency
Abnormally diminished ability of the immune system to resist infection.

Immune suppression
Suppression of the body's resistance.

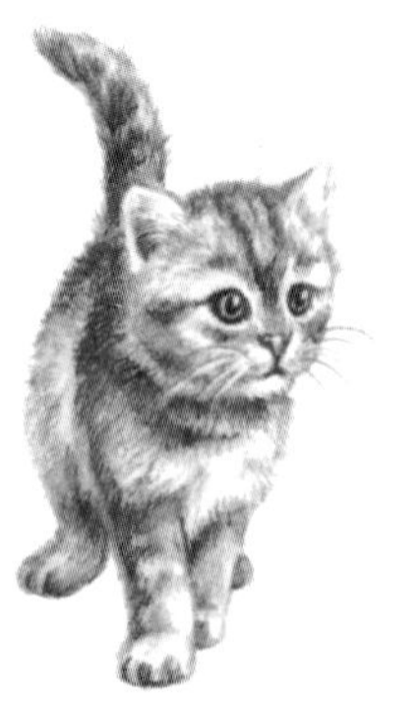

Inbreeding
Mating of related animals. The closer the relationship, the greater the degree of inbreeding. The mating of siblings is the closest degree of inbreeding.

If the parent animals carry concealed detrimental genes, inbreeding results in the more frequent appearance of animals that inherit such bad genetic traits from both parents. Damage caused by inbreeding is the result. By the same token, however, inbreeding can also produce animals that inherit from related parents a genetic trait that breeders desire. In this way inbreeding with genetically sound animals can also serve to reinforce and spread traits desirable to breeders.

Incubation period
Time from contagion until the appearance of the first symptoms of disease.

Infusion
Administering of large amounts of fluid containing electrolytes (see *Electrolytes*), glucose, and other substances. Usually administered intravenously.

Injection
Giving of drugs with the help of a hypodermic syringe and a needle; for example: into the vein (intravenous), under the skin (subcutaneous), into the muscle (intramuscular).

Insecticides
Agents that kill insects.

Intestinal flora
Normal bacteria present in the intestines that are important for healthy digestion.

Killed vaccine
Vaccine with pathogens that have been killed.

Kinked tail
A kinked tail is caused by a malformation of the caudal vertebra. At one time it was considered the hallmark of Siamese cats. Today the kinked tail is considered a serious fault, and it means that the animal will not be used for breeding.

Kneading
Young kittens that are still being nursed by their mother use their front paws to "knead" her teats in order to stimulate the flow of milk. Adult cats also retain this "treading" behavior (for example, to express their well-being to their human).

Lethal factor
Pathological genetic trait that leads to death. With homozygosis (identical pairs of genes), the lethal factor in the genes of the tailless Manx cat results in the death of the fetus.

Life expectancy
With good care indoor cats can live to be fifteen, some-

times even twenty, years old. Free-roaming cats, on the other hand, have a far shorter life expectancy because they frequently fall victim to street traffic or infectious diseases.

Live vaccine
The pathogens of the vaccine are modified in such a way that they still can multiply, but they no longer possess disease-causing properties.

Luxation
Dislocation.

Masked cats
The dark facial marking of a cat breed is called the mask. It contrasts clearly with the rest of the coat. Examples are the Siamese, Birman, and color-point Persian.

Metabolism
Continuous conversion of the body's substances by exchange with substances from the environment.

Metastases
Appearance of tumors at various sites in the body as a result of the spread from a primary tumor.

Mutation
Suddenly occurring change in a genetic substance that results in a change in the cat's color, coat, or build. The genetic trait may be passed on to the offspring.

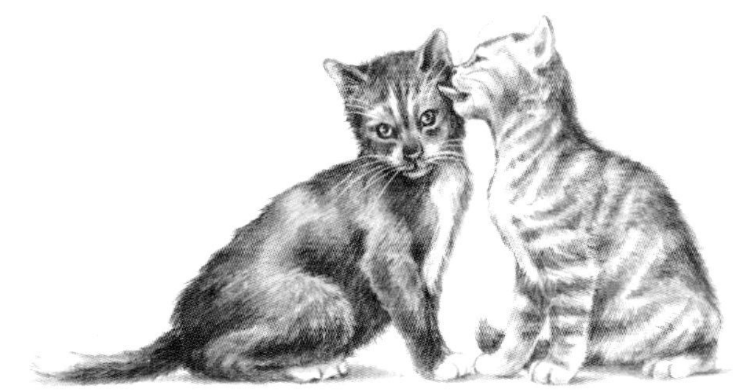

These two cats like each other. Licking the coat is a proof of affection.

Necrosis
Death of body tissue.

Nematodes
Threadworms or roundworms that can attack the cat's intestines.

Nictitating membrane
Third eyelid, which is visible primarily in the event of illness.

Oocysts
Egglike products of the propagation of one-celled parasites.

Ophthalmoscope
Special lamp for examining the area at the back of the eye.

Otoscope
Instrument for observing the auditory canal in the ear.

Ovulation
Release of the egg. It is triggered 25 to 36 hours after mating. Only then does the mature egg leave the ovaries, and it is fertilized, if it is going to be fertilized at all, one to two days later.

Palpation
Examination of the cat by touch.

Panleukopenia
Sharp decrease in the number of white corpuscles in the blood. Feline panleukopenia is known as FPL.

Paramunity inducers
Substances that increase nonspecific resistance to pathogens (for example, the substance used to treat FeLV disease, discussed on page 106).

Physiology of nutrition
The theory of metabolic processes in connection with nutrition.

Praziquantel
Medication used to control tapeworms.

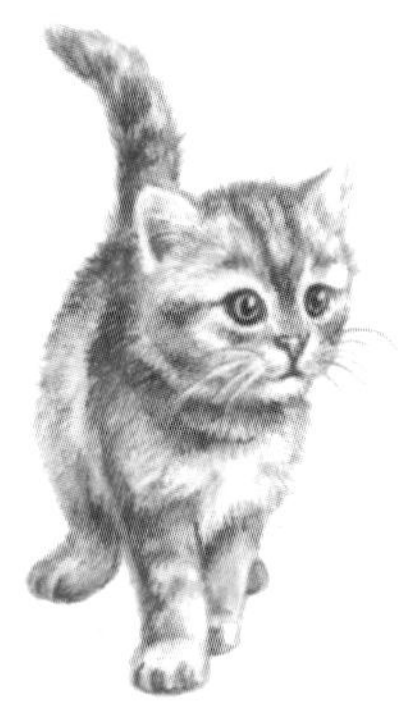

Prior immunity
State of equilibrium between the remaining pathogens and the resistance of the host organism.

Progesterone
A sex hormone that is used to suppress estrus in cats.

Prostaglandins
Special tissue hormones that are administered, for example, when a cat has a uterine infection (see page 82).

Protozoans
One-celled creatures, some of which are parasites.

Purebred (pedigreed) cat
A cat descended from cats systematically bred in order to conform in appearance to a breed standard.

Pyoderma
Skin inflammation caused by bacteria.

Q

Quarantine
Isolation of diseased cats or cats suspected of being contagious. When you take your cat along on vacation, you need to know that some countries, including England, Malta, Australia, New Zealand, Ireland, Norway, and Sweden, require a six-month quarantine for cats because of the danger of rabies. Consequently, you cannot take your pet to those countries on vacation.

R

Radiograph
A photographic image produced by the action of x-rays or nuclear radiation.

Resistance
Immunity of the body to certain harmful factors, or of a disease-causing organism to a medication.

Resorption
Intake of substances into the systemic circulation.

Right to dispense medicines
The veterinarian's privilege of preparing medicines, keeping them on hand, and dispensing them to treat patients.

S

Scent marks
To mark their territory, male cats use urine to leave signals on trees, walls, fences, or furniture. When they spray urine, the animals usually stretch their hind legs to their full height and, with their tails stiffly erect and trembling convulsively, point their hindquarters at the object and direct their spray toward it at an upward angle. Indoors, the smell lingers a very long time, and for this reason it is virtually impossible to keep an uncastrated male indoors.

Individual scent marks can also be left by the secretions of the cheek and anal glands as well as the balls of the feet.

Sclera
Fibrous white skin that surrounds the eyeball.

Secondary infection
A second infection—by bacteria, for example—following an infection, usually caused by viruses, that has weakened the organism.

Secretion
Substance formed and released by the body.

Serologic examination
Determination of diagnostically important substances—antibodies, for example—in the blood serum.

Serum
Blood plasma (blood replacement) without coagulants.

Sexing
To identify the sex of a cat. In a male cat the distance between the anus and the genital opening is greater than in a female. In males the open-

ing itself is round, in females, oval in shape.

Skin scrapings
Scraping off of skin samples for testing for mites, fungi, or other parasites.

Spasmolytics
Antispasmodics.

Sulfonamides (sulfa drugs)
Medications that inhibit the development and multiplication of bacteria much as antibiotics do.

Systemic
Concerning the entire organism.

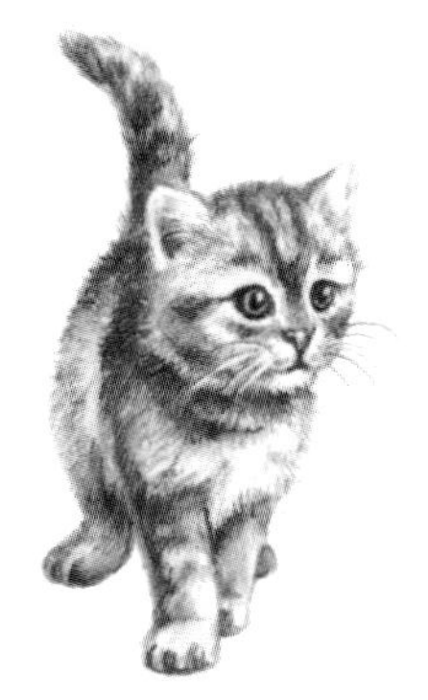

Taurine
An essential amino acid required for the proper development and functioning of the retina and heart.

Teeth
Until their sixth month of life, young cats have 26 milk teeth. An adult can have 30 teeth.

Tetracycline
A medication that is classified as a broad-spectrum antibiotic (see *Broad-spectrum antibiotic*).

Tortoiseshell cat
The name given to cats of three colors—black, red, and cream. The red coloration is linked with the female chromosomes. Tortoiseshell cats are almost always female because of the color genes on the sex chromosomes. Male tortoiseshells are rare and usually sterile.

Toxin
Poisonous substance.

Trauma
Wound, injury, effect of violence; psychological upset.

Ultrasound
Inaudible, high-energy sound waves. Used for diagnostic purposes and for tartar removal, for example.

Uremia
Poisoning of the blood by toxic substances that damaged kidneys are no longer able to remove from the bloodstream.

Vaccination
Inoculation.

Viruses
Simple forms of life that can multiply only with the help of affected cells. Some viruses cause extremely serious diseases in cats.

Zoonosis
Infectious disease that affects humans and animals. Examples are toxoplasmosis and rabies.

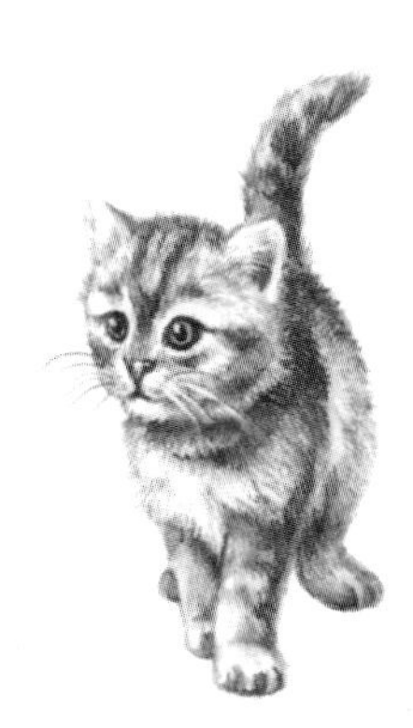

Index

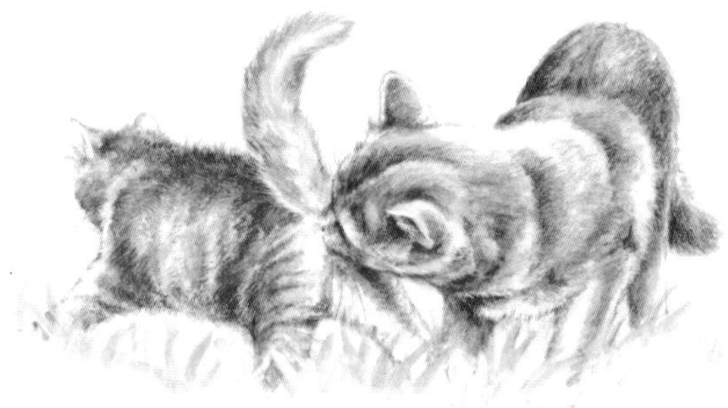

Sniffing to find out whether the kitten is a member of the family.

Information

Useful Reading Materials

For further reading on this subject and related matters, consult the following books also published by Barron's Educational Series, Inc.

Behrend, Katrin, and Wegler, Monika: *The Complete Book of Cat Care,* 1991.
Daly, Carol Himsel: *Caring for Your Sick Cat*, 1994.
Müller, Ulrike: *The New Cat Handbook*, 1984.
Viner, Bradley: *The Cat Care Manual*, 1993.

The following magazines are also very helpful.

Cat Fancy
P.O. Box 6050
Mission Viejo, CA 92690

CATS Magazine
2750-A South Ridgewood Avenue
South Daytona, FL 32119

Popular Cats
1115 Broadway
New York, NY 10010

Animal Behaviorist Referral

Animal Behavior Society
c/o John Wright, Ph.D.
Department of Psychology
Mercer University
1400 Coleman Avenue
Macon, GA 31207

Animal Protection

American Society for the Prevention of Cruelty to Animals (ASPCA)
424 East 92 Street
New York, NY 10128
(212) 876–7700

Homeopathic Veterinary Referral

American Holistic Veterinary Medical Association
2214 Old Emmorton Road
Bel Air, MD 21015

Liability and Health Insurance

Almost all insurance companies now offer liability insurance for pets. Several now also offer health insurance.

The Authors

Hans Alfred Müller has been working in Giessen, Germany, since receiving his degree in veterinary medicine. His fields of specialization include parasitology and behavioral research on domestic animals. He has been a practicing veterinarian for more than ten years, with a great number of cats as patients.

Ulrike Müller has been breeding purebred cats for many years. She has also served as a judge at cat shows in many different countries. In addition, she is the author of three successful pet owner's manuals published by Barron's: *Longhaired Cats* (1984), *The New Cat Handbook* (1984), and *Persian Cats* (1990).

Poisoning Information

In most large cities there are information centers you can call in case of poisoning. Although they are intended for people, you can also call them if your cat is poisoned. Obtain the Poison Control Center telephone number and keep it handy.

The Contributing Author

Heidrun Gratz, a doctor of veterinary medicine, specializes in the holistic treatment of animals.

The Photographers

Christine Steimer has been a free-lance photographer since 1985. She has been specializing in animals since 1989, contributing many photographs to the magazine *Das Tier.*

Other well-known animal photographers have also supplied photos for this book.

The Artist

Renate Holzner is a free-lance illustrator living in Regensburg, Germany. Her broad repertoire includes line drawings, photorealistic illustrations, and computer graphics.

Important Notes

This book is about treating feline diseases. The suggestions and methods of treatment are based on the authors' many years of practical experience. But since every case is different, not every suggestion can have unlimited validity. In spite of the detailed and comprehensive descriptions, the book lays no claim to completeness. That is why it is absolutely necessary to visit the veterinarian if there are complications.

Substances that contain insecticides (see "Baths for Skin Infections," page 52, and "A Home Medical Kit," page 52) have to be handled with great caution. Wearing rubber gloves is recommended, especially for persons with sensitive skin or a tendency to develop allergies.

Some diseases of cats, namely, fungal infection of the skin (page 111), some infectious diseases (such as rabies, page 108), and diseases that are caused by parasites (such as roundworms, page 100, and hookworms, page 101) can be transmitted to humans. Maintain hygienic conditions and, if you suspect a problem, visit your physician. Tell him or her that you have a cat and what disease the cat has.

All cat owners are advised to obtain liability insurance.

Photo Credits

Becker: Pages 104, 105; Cogis/Alexis: Page 109; Cogis/Amblin: Pages 5 top, 81; Cogis/Gissey: Pages 5 bottom left, 65; Cogis/Lanceau: Pages 17, 36, 77; Cogis/Lepage: Page 88; Cogis/Varin: Page 12; Cogis/Vidal: Inside front cover, pages 76, 108; Mahler: Page 71 top, bottom; Muller: Pages 44, 97; Reinhard: Pages 20 top, bottom, 37, 45, 100; Schanz: Front cover; Wegler, Pages 5 bottom right, 40 left, right, 41, 92, 112, 128 top, center, bottom left, inside back cover top left, top right, bottom left, bottom right; Steimer: All other photos.

The title of the German book is *Die Kranke Katze*.
Translated from the German by Kathleen Luft.
First English language edition published in 1995 by Barron's Educational Series, Inc.

Address all inquires to:
Barron's Educational Series, Inc.
250 Wireless Boulevard
Hauppauge, New York 11788

Library of Congress Catalog Card No. 95-9792
International Standard Book Number 0-8120-9136-1

Library of Congress Cataloging-in-Publication Data
Müller, Ulrike.
[Kranke Katze. English]
Healthy cat, happy cat : a complete guide to cat diseases and their treatment / Ulrike and H. Alfred Müller ; contributing author, Heidrun Gratz ; drawings by Renate Holzner and color photos by Christine Steimer and other renowned animal photographers.
p. cm.
Includes index.
ISBN 0-8120-9136-1
1. Cats—Diseases—Treatment. 2. Cats—Health. 3. Homeopathic veterinary medicine. I. Müller, Hans Alfred. II. Title.
SF985.M8513 1995
636.8'089—dc20 95-9792
CIP

PRINTED IN HONG KONG
5678 9955 987654321

Breed-related Problems

Exotic shorthair: Cats with extremely flat Persian-like faces often suffer from tearing eyes (see page 64).

Birman cats: This cat, of a moderate type, has few breed-related hereditary defects.

Scottish fold cat: The typical mark of this breed is its folded ears (see page 67).

Persian cat: Some have constantly tearing eyes (see page 64) and malocclusions (see page 69). Persians have a greater tendency to develop complications during labor because of the large heads of their young (see page 41).

Siamese cats: These purebred cats can suffer from malocclusions (see page 69) and diseases of the retina (see page 67).

Abyssinian cats: Diseases of the retina (see page 67) have been found in these cats, as well as amyloidosis—a life-threatening condition characterized by hard, waxy deposits that can affect several organs.

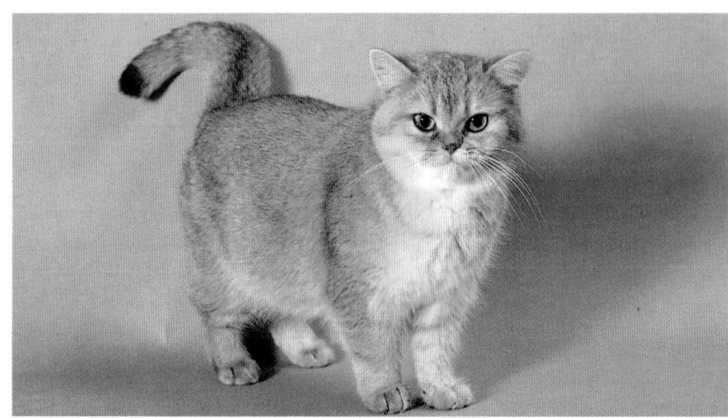

Exotic shorthair

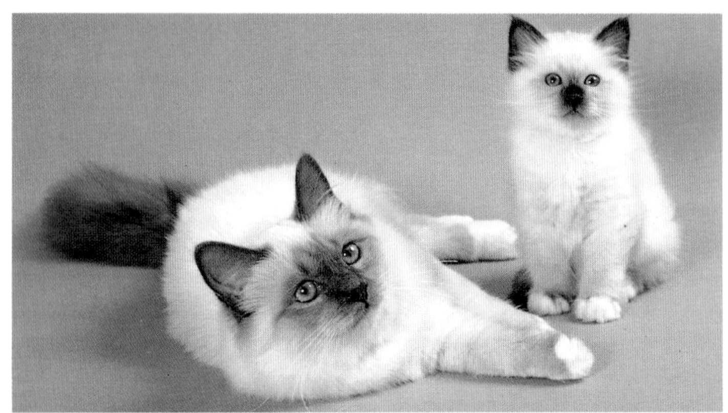

Birman cats

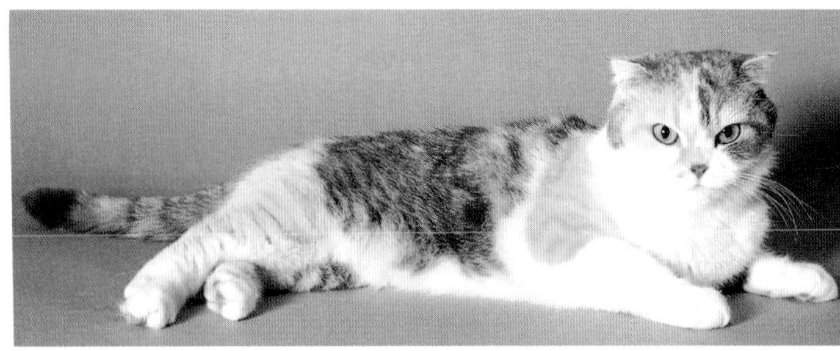

Scottish fold cat

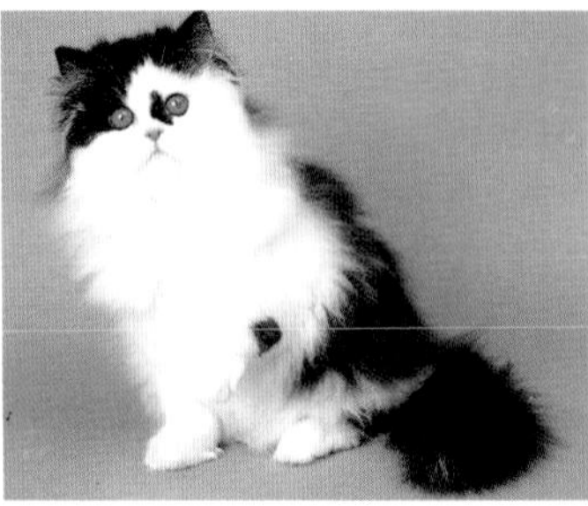

Persian cat